KETOGENIC DIET

The Only Ultimate Keto Diet Blueprint For Beginner
To Start Your Effortless and Permanent Weight Loss

BE FABULOUS!

ROY NOLAN

PAVO
PRESS

Trademarks:

FIRST EDITION

ISBN-13: 978-1-5426-3718-3
ISBN-10: 1-5426-3718-X

Editor: Michelle Gabel
Cover Designer: Annie Eaves
Nutritional Analysis: Isabelle Cruz

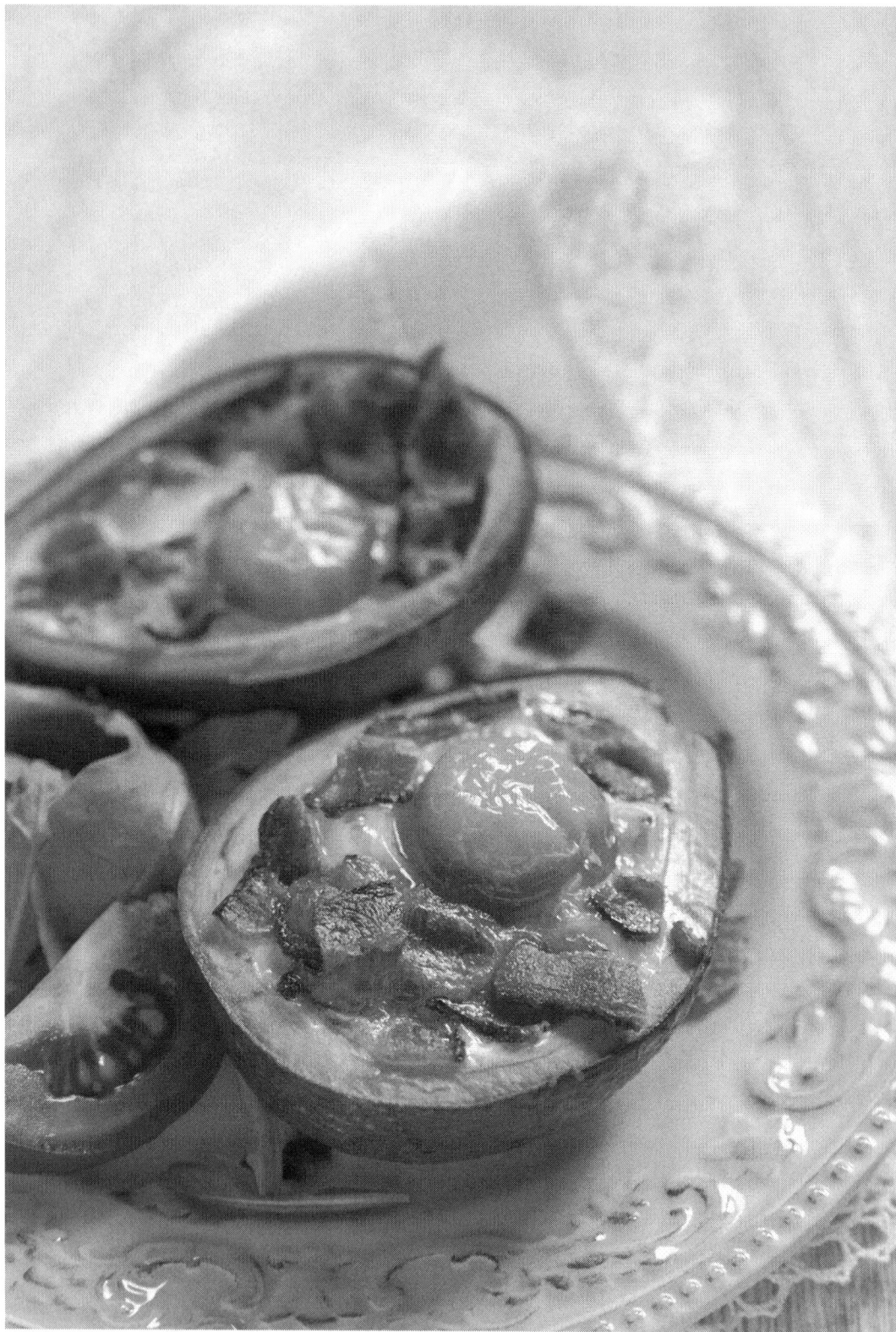

To friendship and to my family,

who make my world more meaningful

CONTENTS

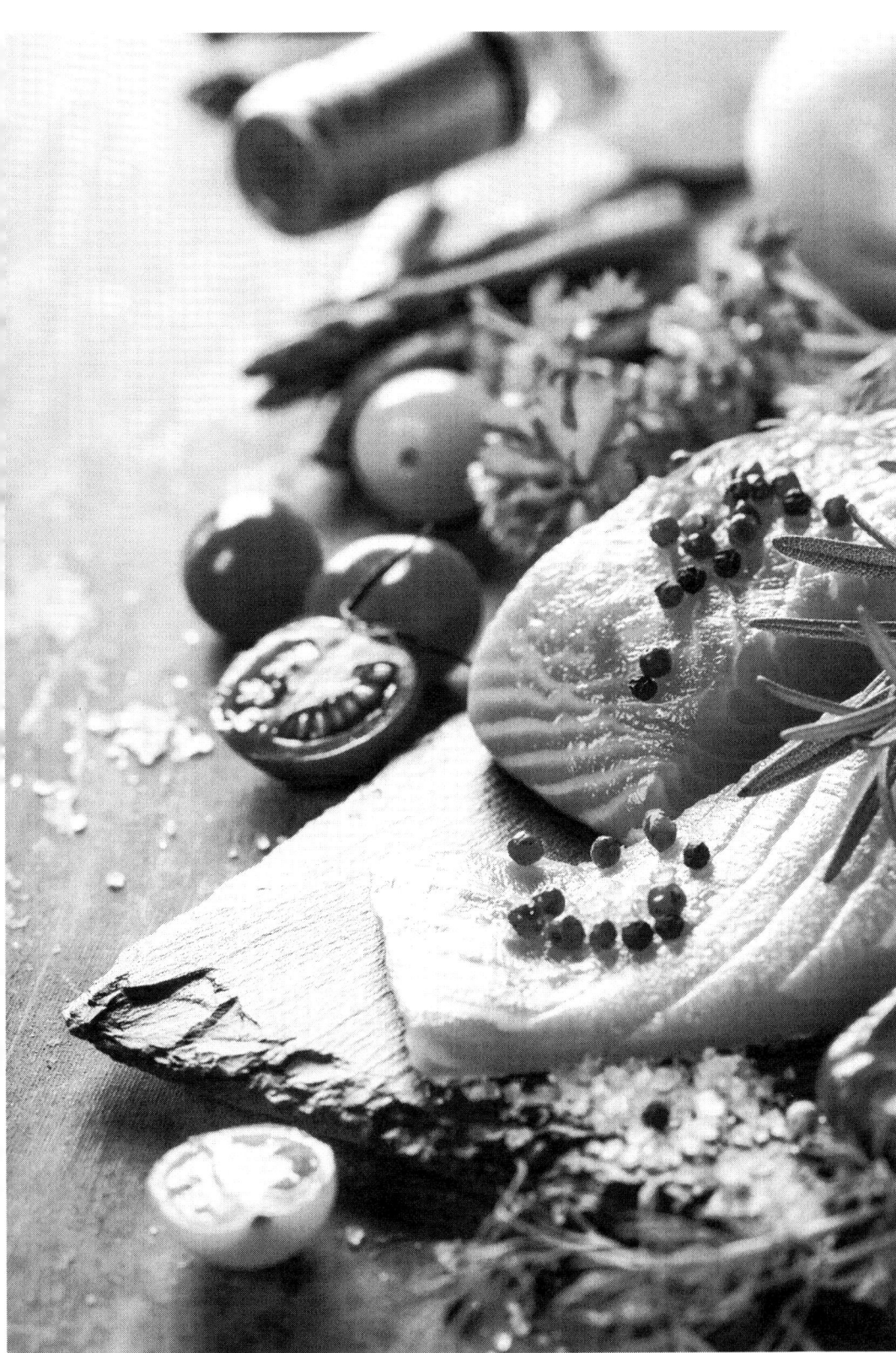

Chapter 1

Introduction

Weight loss. It is a universal goal that connects millions of people worldwide, but a goal that many people give up on before they are able to achieve it.

Let's face it. Weight loss is hard. You must be careful about what you are eating, how much you are eating, and how much activity you get in your day. You have to say "no" to some of the foods you used to indulge in regularly, and you must push at times when you don't feel comfortable to do so.

And to make matters worse, during this time, it seems that the number on the scale doesn't move, and you are suffering for nothing.

I've been there. I know what it's like to try to lose weight and fail. I know how frustrating it is to step on that scale week after week and to see the same number staring back. I was incredibly unhappy and on the verge of giving up on ever being satisfied with my physical appearance.

Then I found the ketogenic diet and it changed my life. Suddenly, I had a meal plan I could stick to, delicious food that I enjoyed eating, and – most importantly- numbers on the scale to back up the diet's efficiency! With the ketogenic diet, I lost over 160 pounds and I feel better than ever.

Now, I want to share this incredible diet plan with you. I want to give you a method that will work and help you lose those pesky pounds you have been trying to eliminate.

You can eat what you want and eat until you feel full. Forget that nagging feeling of hunger. With the ketogenic diet, you can feel satiated at all times while healthily losing weight.

I've tried diets before, and they just didn't work.

I want to lose weight, but I don't have the time to worry about all the foods I can and shouldn't have. There has to be an easier way.

Weight loss has been my goal for months now. I'm tired of being unhappy about how I look, but I don't feel like there's any hope for me.

If you have been struggling to lose weight, thoughts like these are bound to run through your mind. However, don't stress anymore because the solution is here.

This book will provide you with all the answers to any question you might have about the ketogenic diet, and you will find the answers to your weight loss problem.

Learn the basics of the ketogenic diet, practical ways to get started and how to stick with it long term.

You deserve to be happy and love your looks. So, let's get started. Let me show you just how easy this diet is and give you the key to weight loss. You won't believe how fast the weight melts off or how simple losing weight really can be. This book is going to change your life for the better, guaranteed.

Chapter 2

Weight Loss and Healthy Living: Ketogenic Is The Answer

Countless advertisements and devoted followers are enough to convince people to try something new, which is why many start diets that even sound simply absurd.

Although the ketogenic diet also has many dedicated followers, however, unlike other diets, it is highly successful. People all over the world are losing weight – from ten pounds to a couple hundred pounds – all on this same diet.

You know you want these same results and *before* you dedicate all the time and effort to the process, you want to know without a doubt that this diet works.

This is why I will first tell you about the science behind the diet and provide concrete evidence why it works.

The ketogenic diet is a diet that focuses on carbohydrates, fats, and protein. Carbs are to be kept at the bottom of the scale, with fats at the top, and protein in between.

But why do we do things this way?

Nutritionists refer to carbohydrates fats and proteins as macronutrients. These are, in fact, the only three macronutrients which are basically the building blocks of life.

The most important thing is what your body does with the aforementioned nutrients and what makes them crucial for health.

Ironically, most diets recommend consumption of more carbs than other nutrients, which causes weight gain and prevents weight loss. Nevertheless, it's important to understand that not all carbs are the same.

It's difficult to throw a blanket over carbs and label them all as "bad" because there are different kinds of carbs, and your body handles them differently.

When it comes to nutrition, you will hear many people refer to carbs as either "simple" or "complex", though for someone who isn't heavily involved in nutrition it may be easier to think of them as either "whole" or "refined" instead.

As a rule of thumb, healthier foods *do* contain some level of carbohydrates. But, these carbohydrates can be referred to as whole carbs because they are untouched and exactly as found in nature. When you ingest these kinds of carbs, you are also ingesting fiber and other nutrients along.

Whole carbs are found in foods such as vegetables, fruits, whole grains, potatoes, and others in this category. As you can see, this list of foods that is generally considered healthy.

On the other hand, refined carbs are different. These carbs have all nutritional value stripped out of them and all that remains is the carbohydrate itself.

This means you are ingesting pure sugar but nothing good along with it, so your body is going to handle it entirely differently than it would a whole carb. These refined carbs are what tend to spike your blood sugar, then leave you in a crash only minutes later.

If you have ever felt "shaky" or weak after eating refined white carbs, this is the reason why.

Now, these "bad" carbs are found in foods that have been drastically modified, such as white flours, fast foods, processed foods, pre-packaged foods, etc.

White sugar is the worst choice for your body, which is why sweetened fruit juices and sweetened foods are so bad for you.

It's safe to say that refined carbs aren't going to do you any favors and the more you consume them the harder it is going to be for you to lose weight.

It would be nearly impossible to go carb free in your diet because virtually every food contains a certain amount of carbs. However, if you carefully select your food, you can keep this amount to a minimum, pushing your body into ketosis.

Ketosis is a state your body enters when it isn't receiving enough carbs, which it normally burns, from external sources. Due to this lack, your body starts burning the stored fat which results in weight loss.

Your body converts carbs into blood sugar quickly, so the more carbs you put into your body, the more sugar your body can produce. When your body has more sugar than it needs, it stores the rest as fat.

When you cut off the external supply of carbs to your body, it doesn't have any way to create this sugar, so it naturally goes back to its reserves.

Your body also turns protein into sugar, which is why this diet maintains protein at a moderate level.

Protein is essential for health, so it's crucial that you add it to your diet daily. However, too much protein is only going to replace the carbohydrates in your body, preventing you from entering ketosis.

This is a delicate balance, but it's one you can easily achieve with a little practice and effort.

Chapter 3

Getting Facts Straight: What is the Ketogenic Diet?

As you study why the ketogenic diet works and how you can get it to work for you, other questions are sure to arise.

- **What is this diet exactly about?**

- **Where did this diet come from?**

- **How did it gain such popularity?**

- **How can I successfully maintain this diet?**

So, let's answer some questions.

The ketogenic diet is a diet that is primarily low in carbs. If you were to compare it to other diets, this one falls into the low-carb category. However, unlike most low carb diets, the ketogenic diet is a *low carb-high fat,* not a *low carb-high protein diet.*

While on this diet, you can eat virtually anything you want as long as it falls into the low carb/high fat/moderate protein diet.

The ketogenic diet was officially recognized in the 1920s when physicians were experimenting with diets to control epilepsy. They based the diet on the fasting methods of cultures that have used fasting for thousands of years. Some of the most basic rules of the diet can be traced back to methods used by the ancient Egyptians.

Physicians noted that the energy carbohydrates provide were detrimental to patients with epilepsy. By reducing their carb intake, the patients had fewer seizures. However, with the introduction of other medications, this form of treatment became less and less prevalent, until it was only used to treat children who didn't respond well to medication.

As the treatment proved to be effective in children, adults began trying it out and experienced great results. It was soon discovered that this was an effective treatment for a variety of other health ailments... including weight loss.

As the ketogenic diet began to lose popularity for treating epilepsy in lieu of modern medicine, it began to pick up momentum when it came to weight loss. Adults of all ages lost weight easily, even when they struggled with weight loss using other methods.

Of course, when one person sees that a diet works, the word spreads quickly, and soon low carb diets began popping up around the world. However, the ketogenic diet continued to gather many dedicated followers.

When it comes to the diet itself, you may be wondering if there are any specific rules you need to follow.

This diet is remarkably simple when it comes to what you should do to succeed. Instead of focusing on specialty foods or worrying about calories, you simply need to track the intake of fat, protein, and carbs on a daily basis.

In later chapters, I am going to show you the ratios you should follow, which will keep you on track and keep the numbers on the scale going in the right direction.

Chapter 4

A Diet for Everyone?

People come in all shapes and sizes, with their own unique needs. With this in mind, it's important to understand who is able to safely follow the ketogenic diet and who needs to be more conscious of what is going on with their body.

As we saw in the last chapter, the ketogenic diet is often used to treat medical conditions as it has numerous health regulatory capabilities. However, if you are on medication, you must be careful as you start the ketogenic diet as the medication may intensify the effects.

If you are a type 1 or type 2 diabetic, you can start the ketogenic diet but with caution.

Remember that the ketogenic diet is entirely about regulating your blood sugars. If you are using insulin on a regular basis, you have to be extremely careful about the dosage and frequency of your insulin intake.

With careful moderation of your diet, you could potentially get off all medications associated with your diabetes through the ketogenic diet. This is going to require special medical supervision and careful regulation on your part.

It's important to note that those with high blood pressure or who are on blood pressure medications of any kind need to be extremely cautious.

Again, various medications are going to have a more intense effect on your body as it shifts to accommodate your new lifestyle. It is highly advisable continuously to monitor your medication doses and the effects these have on your body as you get used to your new diet.

To minimize side effects, consider taking it slow as you implement your diet. You should not go completely ketogenic overnight, so if you are on any kind of medications take your time and make the transition easy on your system.

Both vegans and vegetarians can also lose weight and enjoy the benefits of the ketogenic diet: they just have to be more creative.

Vegetarians actually won't have to try very hard to start the ketogenic diet, because there are plenty of fat sources found in dairy and eggs. Opt for full-fat milk, a lot of cheese, eggs and, of course, oils.

Though you aren't going to eat any meat products, there are plenty of plant sources of fats. Avocados and nuts are full of fats, so when you combine these with the dairy products, you won't have any problems meeting your fat requirements.

Vegans, on the other hand, need to be a little more creative, though they are going to find that they also have plenty of options from which to choose. When it comes to veganism and the ketogenic diet, you will need to opt for oils.

Familiarize yourself with the use of coconut oil, olive oil, vegetable oil, and any other oils. Calculate the fat content in each one you choose at the time, and consume only as much as daily recommended. Oils are incredibly easy to implement into your diet, so don't worry about meeting the proper ketogenic requirements.

While only you can decide what is right for your body, you need to be cautious during pregnancy.

Whether it is safe or healthy to be on the ketogenic diet while pregnant is a fiercely debated topic. The only right answer is to consult your doctor. While some women stay on the diet the entire duration of their pregnancy, other are able to only stay on the ketogenic diet for a couple months.

If you have any doubts about the diet whatsoever, discuss your concerns with your doctor. Although the ketogenic diet is an incredibly healthy option but when you are pregnant you have someone else to think of, so make sure you are doing what is right for both of you!

For any other conditions, you simply need to monitor how you feel on the new diet. With any medications, pay close attention to the reaction of your body and how you feel as you transition.

The ketogenic diet has proven to be incredibly healthy for people in all stages of life. With the right methods and preparation, you aren't going to have an issue getting on it, either.

Keep in touch with your body and focus on how you feel as you cut your carb intake. Pay attention to how you feel while you lose weight and enjoy the benefits!

Chapter 5

The Process

Now that you know what the ketogenic diet is and whether or not this diet is right for you, it's time to dive into the process. There are several key components in the ketogenic diet and a few separate parts to the process. In this chapter, we are going to discuss each of these parts, and how you can apply them.

If you have done any research on the ketogenic diet prior to reading this book, it's likely you have heard of the 4:1 ratio.

However, unless you have studied further what this means, it is likely you might find it confusing.

In this high fat-low carb diet, you need to focus on the amount of each you are consuming in a day, measured in grams. Now, unlike other diets that keep you under a certain amount of grams per day, your goal is to keep the ratio even.

While you will still need to control your portions the most important thing will be to maintain the proper ratio of the foods you eat. For example, in the 4:1 ratio, you are going to eat 4 grams of fat for every 1 gram of protein and carbs combined.

This means that if you eat a meal that contains 8 grams of fat, you will need to keep the protein and carbs to 1 gram. This can be either 2 grams of protein *or* 2 grams of carbs, or it can be 1 gram of protein *and* 1 gram of carbs, so long as neither one exceeds the ratio of 4:1.

While this sounds really easy to do, and while it is an easy transition to make per se, you may find that you need to take a few extra steps to help transition your metabolism from glucose to fat.

Your body is used to using the fuel you provide it with, so if you have been eating carbs, it's used to running on sugars. When you switch to fat, your metabolism needs time to make this transition.

The first thing you need to remember, as you make this switch in your body, is that fat – not sugar – is your body's preferred source of food.

In ancient times, humankind lived off of nuts, berries, vegetables, meats, and other things that could easily be found. Carbs, and their "bad" counterpart, refined carbs, didn't make an appearance until much later in history.

Nevertheless, you must also remember that your body adapted to a diet high in refined carbs and, therefore, it needs to adapt once more to a diet without them. Whenever your body needs to adapt to anything, it is going to fight you at first.

You may feel tired, you may have a mildly upset stomach, and you may have trouble sleeping when you first start the ketogenic diet. However, keep in mind that these side effects are expected, and temporary.

Your body will adapt to these changes and begin burning the fat it has stored within itself. This is a state referred to as ketosis.

Every nutrient you put in your body is converted into some kind of fuel. You may have heard that protein is the building block of muscles, or felt like fast food goes immediately to your thighs.

This happens because of the way your body treats the food you eat.

When you are on the ketogenic diet, you are depriving your body of carbs, which are quickly changed into sugar. Right now, your body is running on this sugar and feels it needs a constant supply.

Your goal is to teach your body to fuel itself with fat instead of sugar and to do that you simply need to end the supply of carbs. Once you cut off the external supply of carbs, your body will naturally begin looking for another source of fuel.

Some people fear that minimizing carbs intake is going to push the body into starvation mode but trust me - if you are eating fats and proteins, it won't.

Since the ketogenic diet allows you to eat until you are satiated, your body isn't going attack your muscle as it would if you were starving yourself. You are giving your body all the calories you need to function but you aren't giving your body all the carbs it thinks it needs.

As a result, your body burns through the fat reserves it has stored, which is called ketosis.

Chapter 6

Making the Switch

As you become familiar with the ketogenic diet, you will notice the term "the switch" popping up repeatedly. This will likely make you wonder what this alleged switch is and what it means for you.

In this chapter, I want to focus on how you can make this keto switch and what you can expect along the way.

For most people, the keto switch is as easy as switching your diet from food rich in carbs to food that is high in fats and low in carbs.

While you must be careful if you are on any medications, in general, this is going to be exceptionally easy. However, it's quite likely you will experience a few uncomfortable symptoms when you first make the switch. I'll touch deeper on these later on but, for now, simply focus on making the switch quickly and easily.

The hardest part of this process is going to be ignoring the cravings for carbs. Your body knows what it wants and as your supplies run low it's going to be craving them. It will be harder and harder the longer you go without them.

As with all other aspects of life, however, your body is going to adjust to this, too, and with time, the cravings will subside and you'll lose weight.

To make this switch as easy as possible, it's important to understand what you can and can't consume. Of course, this is just a generalized list.

Foods you can freely consume:

- Heavy cream
- Full-fat dairy
- Meats of all kinds
- Butter
- Oils
- Green beans
- Carrots

- Salads

- Most vegetables

- Berries

- Unsweetened fruits

- Bread and pasta substitutes

- Tofu

- Cheese

- Etc.

For each of the foods on this list, you will notice that they are high in fat and moderate in protein while being exceptionally low in carbs. As I mentioned already, not all carbs are equal and the carbs you find in the vegetables and fruits, though minimal, aren't going to affect your body in the same way in which refined white carbs do.

This is why it is also important to avoid sugars and sugar-sweetened food, even if the food would otherwise be fine to consume. As you step into the ketogenic diet, you will learn how to view the whole picture and choose foods you want to eat based on every component.

In other words, you might choose to eat a peach, but you will not choose to eat canned peaches in heavy syrup. The same principle applies to the other foods as well.

Foods you will generally avoid:

- Rice

- Breads

- Potatoes

- Candies

- Pastries

- Crackers

- Chips

- Cereals

- White flour products

- Wheat flour products

- Sweetened juices

- Sodas

- Etc.

As you can see, many of the foods listed here are laden with carbs regardless of their origin. Even certain vegetables, such as potatoes, are full of carbs, though they are on the veggie list.

Again, breaking into the ketogenic diet is going to take some time and practice but with patience and effort, you will have the lists and principles memorized and won't have to think twice about what you are eating.

Though the list of foods to avoid looks rather long and daunting, you would be amazed at how much overlap there is within the categories and the types of foods you can consume on your new diet.

While it will take some time to adjust to some of the foods - especially to the fact that sweets are forbidden -you will be amazed at the speed of your adjustment.

Chapter 7

Reaping The Reward: Ketogenic Diet Benefits

Now it's time to break into one of the most important chapters of the book and give you all the motivation you will ever need to stick with this diet. Keep in mind that various people achieve results at various levels and what you experience may vary compared to other people's experiences.

However, if you stick to the diet for any amount of time, surely you will notice all the changes.

The biggest benefit you will receive from the ketogenic diet is weight loss.

Obviously, this is the goal of this diet, so we will first focus on this benefit. So far I have explained the mechanisms of the ketogenic diet and how it affects your body and contributes to weight loss. I have also explained the possible side effects and what you can expect when you start the diet.

Although this diet was originally noticed to affect various conditions, such as epilepsy, it wasn't long before people all over the world realized that this is an incredibly efficient weight loss tool. By making a few simple changes in your diet, you are able to change your life.

Different people lose weight at a different pace. Therefore, you may find that right from the start you rapidly weight, or you may find that you lose weight slower, but consistently. However, regardless of the speed at which you lose your excessive pounds, rest assured that it will happen and you will reach your weight goal.

The ketogenic diet will help you regulate your blood sugar levels, meaning you won't get that shaky or weak feeling throughout your day.

Nobody likes to feel weak or shaky, or as if they are going to faint. However, for those who are trying to lose weight, this is a very common complaint. The reason many people feel this way when they are trying to lose weight is that their blood sugar plummets between meals.

When you are on the ketogenic diet, your insulin level will be regulated, which means you will feel full, and you will not have to worry about a blood sugar attack sneaking up on you between meals.

Even when you are hungry, your blood sugar isn't going to fall like it used to when you were consuming more carbs and thus you won't get that weak or shaky feeling.

The ketogenic diet has been used to treat and prevent a variety of chronic illness and people who are on this diet don't develop the same illnesses that their carb eating counterparts do.

If you look back in time, chronic diseases were not the same as they are today. People didn't hear of various conditions such as Alzheimer's disease or diabetes as often as they do now, although they did exist.

Obesity wasn't as nearly common as today, and it was not the cause of many underlying health related issues. In fact, the ketogenic diet was used to treat a variety of health issues, starting with epilepsy. To this day, this diet is recommended for a wide range of illnesses. Moreover, it is rare that people on this diet develop chronic illnesses.

Even if you are on this diet only to lose weight, you can be sure you are doing more for your health than you would be if you were to start any other diet.

If there is one thing you hear many people complain about, it is the lack of focus. The ketogenic diet ensures better clarity of the mind and better focus throughout the day.

Your mind will benefit from the ketogenic diet for several reasons.

For starters, your brain is largely made up of fats. It thrives on glucose, a form of sugar derives from carbs for the brain to function actively. With the reduction of carbs intake in ketogenic diet, the brain will have to look for alternative source of energy to fuel its cellular activities.

The brain is not able to use fat directly for energy. It relies on the liver to generate the ketone bodies primarily from the fatty acids in your ketogenic diet or body fat. These ketone bodies will be the partial replacement fuel for the brain when glucose is insufficient as the primary fuel.

This metabolic state is also known as the Ketosis where some of the body's energy supply is sourced from the ketone bodies in the blood.

What does this means to you?

The more fat you are putting into your body, the better your brain is able to function. Though your body gets used to using carbs, your brain doesn't run on carbs, but on ketone bodies from your body fat and fatty acids in your diet.

This will moves you another step forward and creates a better chance in your effort for weight loss.

Therefore, when you are giving your brain the nutrients it needs, you can expect to be more alert, to have a brighter outlook on your day, and better focus throughout.

Secondly, if you really give it some thought, you will realize that you lose focus when you are hungry. That weak and shaky feeling takes over and all you can think about is the lunchtime.

When you are on the ketogenic diet, you are never going to experience a shaky feeling, meaning you can stay focused throughout your whole day getting your work completely done between meals.

Besides gaining certain benefits in mental clarity and weight loss, you will also notice an increase in your energy levels.

Again, this is directly tied to the amount of sugars you are consuming. When you are eating sugar, your blood sugar will spike and you will feel as though you have energy but this is short term.

Your blood sugar is going to crash, and you will be left feeling tired and craving more sugar. But, when you are on the ketogenic diet, you are not going to experience this spike, which also means you are not going to have to deal with a crash.

Instead, your body is going to work through a steady stream of energy, giving you what you need to get through your day without having to stop and pick yourself up again. Though it's going to take a few days for your body to build up energy, you aren't going to miss the crashes, trust me.

These are just a few of the many benefits you will experience when you are on the ketogenic diet.

People who have gone on this diet have reported feeling better overall. They don't take as much time to fall asleep, they sleep better and reach a deeper level of sleep.

This diet is excellent for immunity and an addition to fighting off the chronic illnesses many people face. The diet will also help your short-term health by keeping your body balanced and immunity strong.

Few things suppress your immunity like white flour and sugar, and when you are on a diet that is high in carbs, it is almost certain you are consuming a lot of both. When on the ketogenic diet, you are not consuming any of the unhealthy things but you are filling your body with nutrients that are actually beneficial, which leads to a stronger immune system.

At the end of the day, while on the ketogenic diet, there are only a few things you aren't going to enjoy. Get started as soon as you can and start enjoying these benefits yourself!

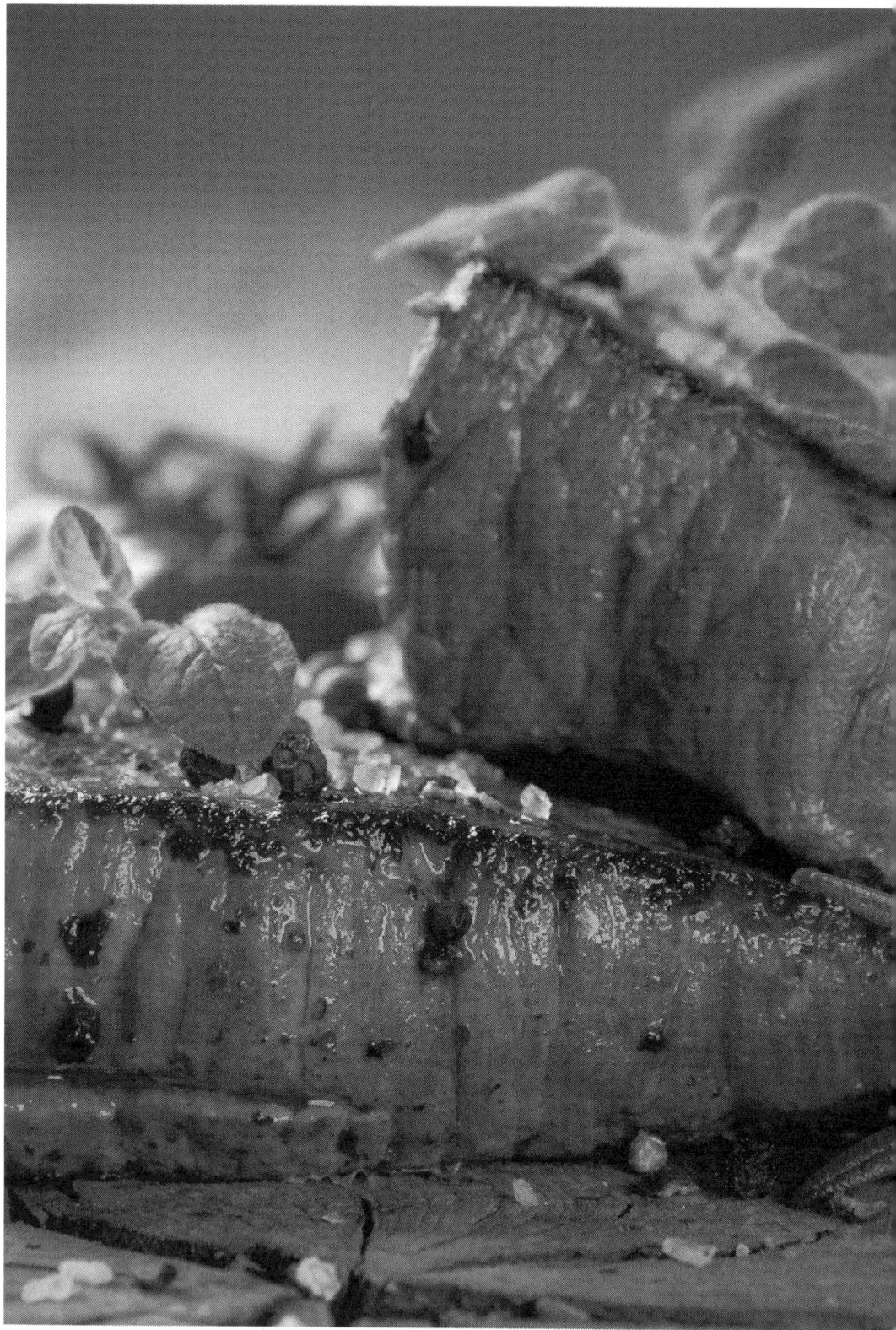

Chapter 8

A Discussion on Ketosis

As you know, the entire goal of the ketogenic diet is to get into a state known as ketosis. Ketosis occurs when your body stops looking for carbohydrates from external sources and begins burning the fat reserves you have stored.

This happens when your body burns fat and not muscle. Only then, you can lose weight effectively, without having to do a lot of extra work, which is usually required when on other types of diet. All you should do is pay attention to the amount of carbs, protein, and fat levels. Remember that the key is eating low amounts of carbs and high amounts of fat.

It is important to understand there is a difference between ketosis and ketoacidosis.

Ketosis is when your body starts burning the fat accumulated inside the body and is entirely different from ketoacidosis, which I will explain later.

The entire reason you lose weight on the ketogenic diet is because you enter ketosis. The goal of the diet is to get your body into this state and while you will get there by eating small amounts of carbs and larger amounts of fat, you have to understand that it takes dedicated practice to get there.

At first, your body is going to fight your decision not to eat carbs and you will have to maintain a steady commitment to your goal.

The cravings are going to seem really intense, especially at first, but you'll get there. One of the benefits of ketosis is that you can reach it in only a few days and once you have, you will experience a brief state of accelerated weight loss.

This is going to taper off after a week or so but after that, you can expect consistent weight loss week by week.

How do I know if I have entered ketosis?

There are several symptoms of ketosis that are unmistakable. Ketosis is one of those things that doesn't require you to guess. If you are experiencing these symptoms, you are likely in the state – especially if you are losing weight.

- **Fruity tasting or bad breath** – acetone is partially removed from your body through your breath and when this is happening in greater amounts than it normally does you can expect a fruity tasting breath or a bad breath as a result.

- **Weight loss** – I've already run through the many reasons you will lose weight when on this diet and weight loss it's by far one of the greatest things you will look forward to when you give up your carbs.

- **Increased ketones in your blood** – again, ketones are always running through your body and you can measure them in your blood, breath, or urine. If you have a breath analyzer, you will be able to keep track of the ketones in your blood without even needing to prick your skin.

- **Increased ketones in your breath or urine** – again, you can keep track of the ketones in your body using a breath analyzer, which you can find in many health stores, department stores, or online.

- **More focus and energy** – It's amazing how well your brain responds to running on fat and not sugars or carbs.

- **Feeling less hungry than normal** – This isn't at all a bad thing, especially if you are trying to lose weight. When you are on the ketogenic diet, you aren't going to have blood sugar spikes or falls, which means you aren't going to have to worry about feeling hungry – or hungry between meals.

- **Bouts of fatigue** – As your body adjusts to the new way of metabolizing your food, you may feel tired. Though this is annoying, it's a sign that you are on the right track with your ketogenic diet.

- **Bouts of lesser performance during your day –** Again, this is a result of your body trying to adjust to your new way of eating. Within a few days, it will wear off and you will be back to your old self in no time.

- **Insomnia –** Some people feel fatigued, others can't sleep. When it comes to ketosis, you cannot always be sure what you are going to experience. However, insomnia, within the first few days of giving up carbs, is a good sign and you are on the right track.

- **Digestive issues –** It isn't at all uncommon to feel an upset stomach, especially at first. Stick with it, drink plenty of water and let your body adjust. It's not fun to go through this but you are going to feel so much better when it's over – even better than ever before.

It's likely when you first start your ketogenic journey, you are going to meet people who are concerned about the effects of ketosis and who claim that it is unhealthy. However, these people are actually referring to ketoacidosis, a dangerous disease.

If you are on the ketogenic diet, it is important that you understand what are ketosis and ketoacidosis, as well as the difference between the two. While you want to enter ketosis, it is important that you do not enter ketoacidosis. If you experience any of the symptoms, immediately make the necessary adjustments.

Ketoacidosis is a diabetic condition in which your body doesn't develop enough insulin. You will not get this condition from the ketogenic diet, however, anyone with the condition will feel it's symptoms, regardless of the other things they have going on in life.

More often than not, the diagnosis of ketoacidosis goes hand in hand with a type 1 diabetes diagnosis and it has nothing to do with the ketogenic diet.

Fainting, weakness, vomiting, and other severe symptoms are present with ketoacidosis. If you are experiencing these symptoms, it is important that you head to the hospital immediately and seek medical help.

If you ever hear anyone say that you need to be careful with the ketogenic diet because of ketosis, they are likely confusing the two conditions and assuming the worst. It is best to not get drawn into any kind of argument but to rather allow them to have their opinion, or to gently inform them of the difference between the two conditions and explain what you are doing.

As long as you understand what ketosis is, and you are careful to monitor your symptoms, you are going to end up with the results you want.

Now, let's get back to ketones. What are they? What is ideal? And how can you make sure you are in the right range?

Just as your body turns carbs into sugar, your body turns fat into ketones. Instead of running on sugar or glucose as it once did, your body is now going to run on ketones.

It's important that you understand how many ketones you want in your body at a time, and how to control that range. As with glucose and insulin, ketones are measured in your blood.

Full ketosis takes place at 1.5-3 mmol/L, and this is what you want your body to be close to most of the time. You can enter ketosis at 0.5 mmol/L quite early on but for the best results, you want to enter full ketosis.

Keep an eye on your ketone level through testing strips using a needle, much like people with diabetes test for insulin; you can also use urine strips. There are even breath analyzers you can purchase, which will last for a long time.

Of the three, I recommend spending the money and getting the breath analyzer. Though the strips are far less expensive, you do have to buy them frequently, depending on how often you test. With the analyzer, all you need to do is pay the up-front fee and you are set.

Decide which the right is for you and stick with that. You can even try various methods to find the one that works, just make sure you are happy and comfortable with your method and that you can stick with it frequently.

As you remain on the ketogenic diet, you are going to measure your ketone level often, even after you have been on the diet for some time. At first, you are going to get an idea of the changes that are taking place in your body but the more you progress with the diet, the easier it will be to keep track.

Now, let's get started with our study of the keto ratio, and your meal plan.

Chapter 9

The Keto Ratio

I have already lightly touched on what the keto ratio is, and why it is important for you to have it in your ketogenic diet. Though most people choose to have the 4:1 ratio, another common ratio you see is the 3:1.

I recommend the 4:1 ratio as that is really easy to follow and keep track of, though it is always best to find what works for you and stick with that. The entire success of this diet rests on whether you enjoy what you are doing and feel as though you can stick with it, so don't hesitate to try out a few different methods.

As you know, the ratio of your nutrients intake is the most important thing in your diet. In the 4:1 ratio, you

are going to consume 4 parts fat to 1 part carbs and protein combined.

Naturally, in the 3:1 ratio, you will be doing the same with the fats and protein, only you will be eating more fats compared to the protein than otherwise. Again, this just comes down to your own preference, and once you decide what you want to do, you can move on to measuring your foods.

If it helps, use a calculator and a journal to keep track of your day to day consumption and progress.

Keeping an eye on your ratios is surprisingly easy if you know how.

The entire ketogenic diet is based on building blocks and cycles that interact with each other. Your first goal is to cut down on the carbs and focus on the fats and moderate protein intake.

You can keep an eye on the ketosis you are in through the various symptoms you feel and you can confirm your progress and range through the strips or analyzer of your choice.

At that point, decide what ratio you wish to use. Calculate the ratio you are eating based on the ingredients in the food you consume. If you look for recipes that are ketogenic friendly, you are likely going to encounter the exact amount of grams fat, protein, and carbs have in every particular product.

It is your job to keep track of all this information as you enjoy the ketogenic diet, but you don't have to do it alone.

There are countless online resources for those who are on the ketogenic diet, from online calculators and food journals to groups and pages dedicated to the diet. Once you decide what is right for you, you can start the diet.

In the next chapter, I am going to tell you more about this ratio, and how you can use it to choose the optimal meal plan for yourself. In no time at all, you are going to start losing weight, on your way to ketosis, enjoying all of the wonderful ketogenic benefits.

Chapter 10

14 Days Starter Meal Plan

You have learned a lot about the ketogenic diet, from how and why it works to all the things you can expect to happen when you yourself start the journey. Now, it is time to stop talking about the diet, and start living it.

In this chapter, I am going to provide you with necessary information about your first 2 weeks on the ketogenic diet, giving you the push you need to change your life.

As we have already discussed and mentioned several times, you need to keep track of the fats to carbs ratios you are putting into your body. You can do this in several different ways.

Most people calculate the amount of fats compared to the amount of carbs and proteins they are eating per meal. This is a fast and easy way to keep track of what you are putting in your body, and will keep you on track with the diet overall.

For starters, it is important to understand that you will measure the amounts in grams rather than calories. Though many weight loss experts will tell you to count calories, calories are going to do you a real disservice here.

Fat is measured in much higher calories than carbs, so comparing the two is going to give you a different outcome than the weight of the two. A single gram of fat is going to weigh the same as a single gram of protein or carbs, so your ratio is precisely 4:1.

If you were to break this down into percentages, you want 80% of your diet to be fat, if you are comparing the ratio by weight. If you are comparing calories, however, you want 90% of your caloric intake to be from fats.

As I said in chapter 5, this is important because fat is much better processed than sugars and used as fuel. I want to explain this process better now, to provide a thorough understanding of how it all works.

When you are eating too many carbs – which is more than the minimal amount a day – your metabolism is going to tear through it. It is going to turn most of the fuel directly into fat and store it in places you don't want.

Your body is also used to doing things in moderation. That means that intake of too many carbs too quickly will end up your body processing a lot of fat all at once. This glucose is also the culprit behind producing what is known as glycerol-3-phosphate, a substance that can be easily referred to as "fixed fats" because it is hard for your body to lose it once it has been formed.

To make matters worse, as you are eating more carbs, you aren't going to be releasing any fat from your body.

As you can see, the more carbs and sugars you eat, the more the weight piles on and the more it resist to come off again.

This sparks a vicious cycle in your body because sugars also make you feel hungry. The more sugars you eat, the hungrier you feel and the more you will crave sugars. This leads to the process starting all over again and leads to the development of more weight problems.

However, when you switch to a diet which is high in fats and low in carbs, your body learns to burn the fats but at a much slower pace.

As we already saw, fats are more calorically dense than carbs, so it will take fewer fats to keep you full than carbs would.

Additionally, it is important to note that your metabolism processes carbs at a lower rate, so you aren't going to feel hungry soon after eating.

Your body also uses fats for fuel. Practically, this means your body is going to burn the fat you eat, and will not store it. As you saw in the previous section, the more carbs you eat – which turn into sugars – the more fat is stored. However, when you are eating fats in the first place, your body is going to burn the fat without storing any.

Therefore, your metabolism learns to burn fats and turns to using itself as a source of energy.

As your body adapts to this new lifestyle, you will find that your energy increases, you sleep better, you have greater focus and, most importantly, you lose weight. But, as with every good thing, there is some degree of discomfort. Before I let you go, I want to show you what some of the most common physical effects are.

Remember that your body needs time to adjust to this new diet and there are going to be a few unpleasant reactions you may experience at first.

These are just temporary and will clear up within a few days to a couple of weeks.

These effects can include:

- Vomiting, diarrhea, upset stomach

- Headaches

- Dizziness and nausea

- Insomnia

- Body odor

- Temporary pauses in weight loss

- Keto rashes

As I said, these things are temporary and will wear off with time. Stick with the diet and be patient as you work through these unpleasant effects. You will find out soon that these side effects subside and you will start feeling a lot better.

Then, the weight will start to come off and you will experience a plethora of other benefits from the diet.

Remember that pairing diets with an exercise regimen is always the healthiest way to lose weight and that with consistency and dedication you will accomplish your goal in no time!

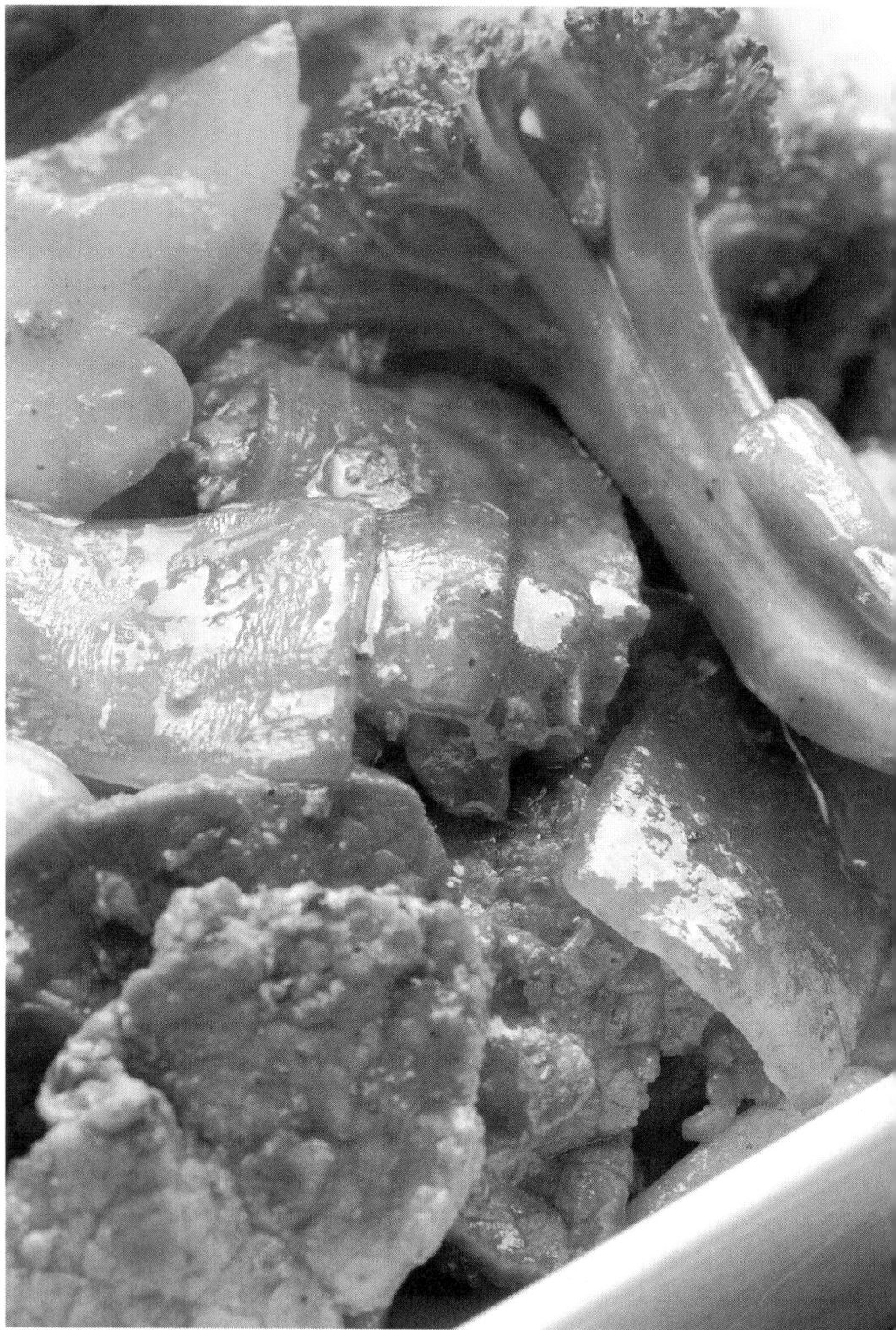

This will be your first week in starting your ketogenic diet. Your body may starts reacting to the keto diet meal routine and you will probably experience some side effects. These are just passing clouds and it will get better. What you will be experiencing is known as the keto-adapt period and everyone has slightly different symptoms and some are shared earlier in this chapter.

For this week, the objective is to kickstart your keto-adaption without the harshness and reduce or softening these unpleasant reactions.

It is recommended to go with the standard ketogenic diet (SKD) first. The SKD consists of

- 70% of high fat
- 25% of moderate protein
- 5% of low carbohydrate

You are looking at about 20 – 30 grams of daily carbohydrate intake.

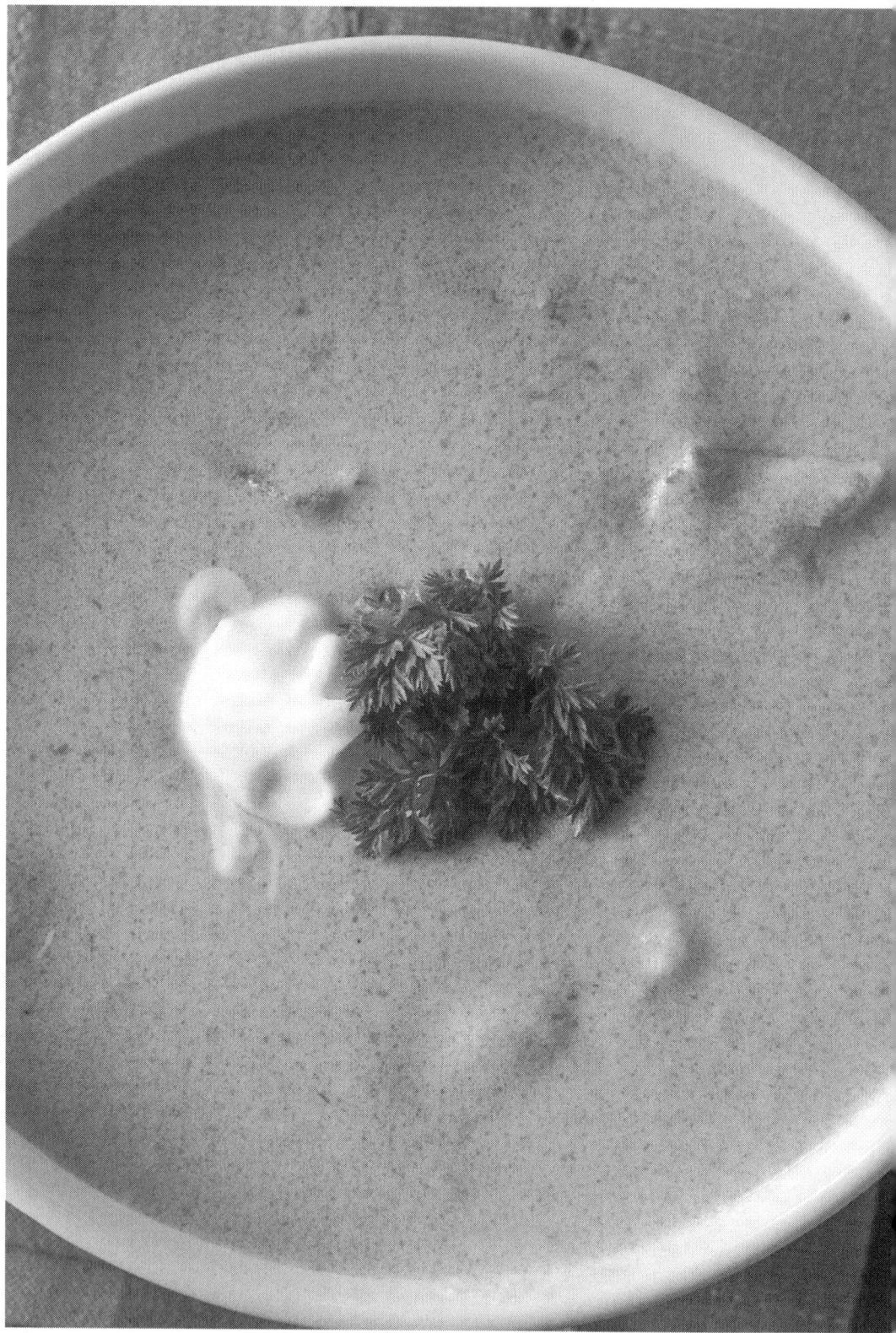

Day 1 Meal Plan

Breakfast	*All-in Omelet*
Snack	*Pepper Sea Salt Pork Rinds*
Lunch	*Roasted Chicken Thighs*
Dinner	*Beefy Tacos*
Dessert	*Coconut Oil Candies*

Day 2 Meal Plan

Breakfast	*Ketogenic Pancakes*
Snack	*Cheesy Bacon Wrap Sticks*
Lunch	*Spinach Stuffed Pork Chops*
Dinner	*Baked Chicken in Creamy Herb Sauce*
Dessert	*Mint Fudge*

Day 3 Meal Plan

Breakfast	*Bread-Free Sandwich*
Snack	*Homemade Chicken Nuggets*
Lunch	*Slow cooked Lobster Bisque*
Dinner	*Roasted Veg and Egg*
Dessert	*Keto Lemon Curd*

Day 4 Meal Plan

Breakfast	*Heavenly Cups*
Snack	*Double Chocolate Chip Cookies*
Lunch	*Easy Salmon with Avocado*
Dinner	*Ribeye Steak in Wild Mushroom*
Dessert	*Cardamon Shortbread Cookies*

Day 5 Meal Plan

Breakfast	*Cheesy Sausage Pie*
Snack	*Fried Avocado with Lemon*
Lunch	*Salmon Fillets*
Dinner	*Chicken and Parmesan Patties*
Dessert	*Keto Avocado Pudding*

Day 6 Meal Plan

Breakfast	*Egg and Avocado Salad*
Snack	*Hard Boiled Egg*
Lunch	*Hearty Chicken Soup*
Dinner	*Beef Stir-Fry*
Dessert	*Ginger Spice Cookies*

Day 7 Meal Plan

Breakfast	*Full-Plate Breakfast*
Snack	*Keto Meatballs*
Lunch	*Beef Balls in Creamy Sauce*
Dinner	*Chicken Filled Zucchini Boats*
Dessert	*Coconut Pudding*

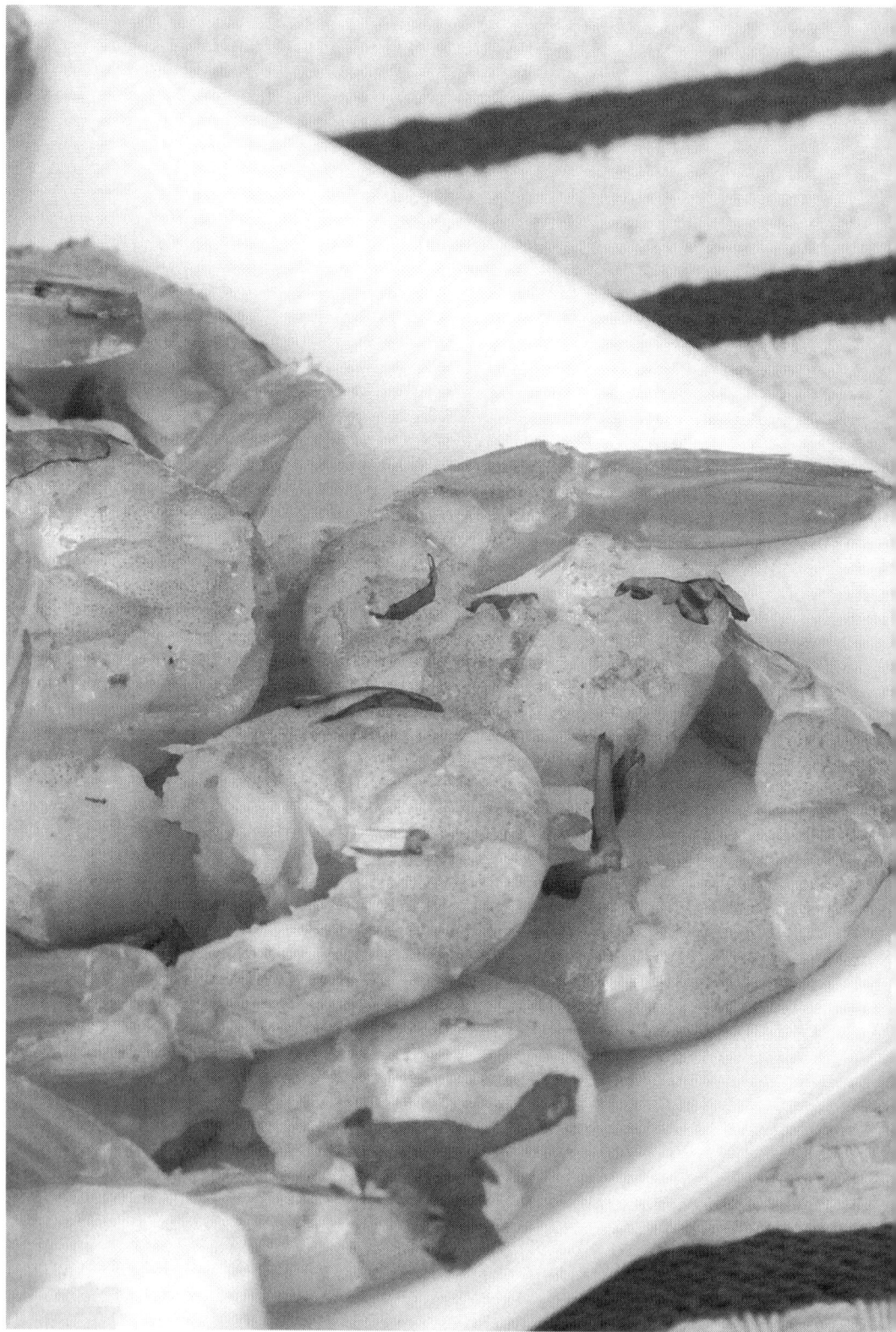

In this week, the objective is to continue your keto-adaption process and once you are keto-adapted (which can usually take a few weeks to a month depending on individuals body conditions), it will be a second nature for your body to accommodate ketone bodies as the body fuel for your daily activities. This will be the beginning of your effortless and permanent weight loss journey.

What if it takes more than two weeks for you to be keto-adapted?

Don't panic. It is very common and you will just need to stay faithful to the keto diet and make sure that you are following the SKD diligently, avoid any bad habits and repeat the meal plan. You will see results very soon.

Day 8 Meal Plan

Breakfast	*Keto-Friendly Porridge*
Snack	*Double Chocolate Chip Cookies*
Lunch	*Parmesan Crusted Fish*
Dinner	*Slow Cooked Spicy Chicken*
Dessert	*Low Carb Cheesecake Brownies*

Day 9 Meal Plan

Breakfast	*Pesto and Eggs*
Snack	*Keto Meatballs*
Lunch	*Buttered Shrimp*
Dinner	*Beefy, Gooey Cheese, Goodness*
Dessert	*Mint Fudge*

Day 10 Meal Plan

Breakfast	*All-in Omelet*
Snack	*Fried Avocado with Lemon*
Lunch	*Slow-Cooked Herbed Beef*
Dinner	*Fish in Orange Pecan Butter Sauce*
Dessert	*Keto Peanut Butter Popsicles*

Day 11 Meal Plan

Breakfast	*One Pan Breakfast*
Snack	*Salted Crispy Macadamia Nuts*
Lunch	*Baked Sardines*
Dinner	*Filet Mignon Steak*
Dessert	*Keto Avocado Pudding*

Day 12 Meal Plan

Breakfast	*Bread-Free Sandwich*
Snack	*Pepper Sea Salt Pork Rinds*
Lunch	*Beef Sausage and Bacon Pot*
Dinner	*Creamy Shrimp and Bacon Bowl*
Dessert	*Ginger Spice Cookies*

Day 13 Meal Plan

Breakfast	*Egg and Avocado Salad*
Snack	*Granola Bars*
Lunch	*Pork Skewers*
Dinner	*Tuna Salad*
Dessert	*Keto Almond Coffee Ice Cream*

Day 14 Meal Plan

Breakfast	Cheesy Sausage Pie
Snack	Crunchy Kale Chips
Lunch	Aloha Burger
Dinner	Salmon and Avocado Omelet
Dessert	Yummy Brownies

SUMMARY

The 14 days meal plan is to guide and assist you in your keto-adaption period. Some may need just a week and other may take more than a few weeks to be keto-adapt.

What's next?

Good question!

After you have become keto-adapt. Congrats! You can still follow or use the keto diet recipes in this book. You may need to move away from the standard ketogenic diet and adopt a more aggressive approach.

Always do your research and read more relevant books to boost your current progress and be on a fast track route to your permanent weight loss.

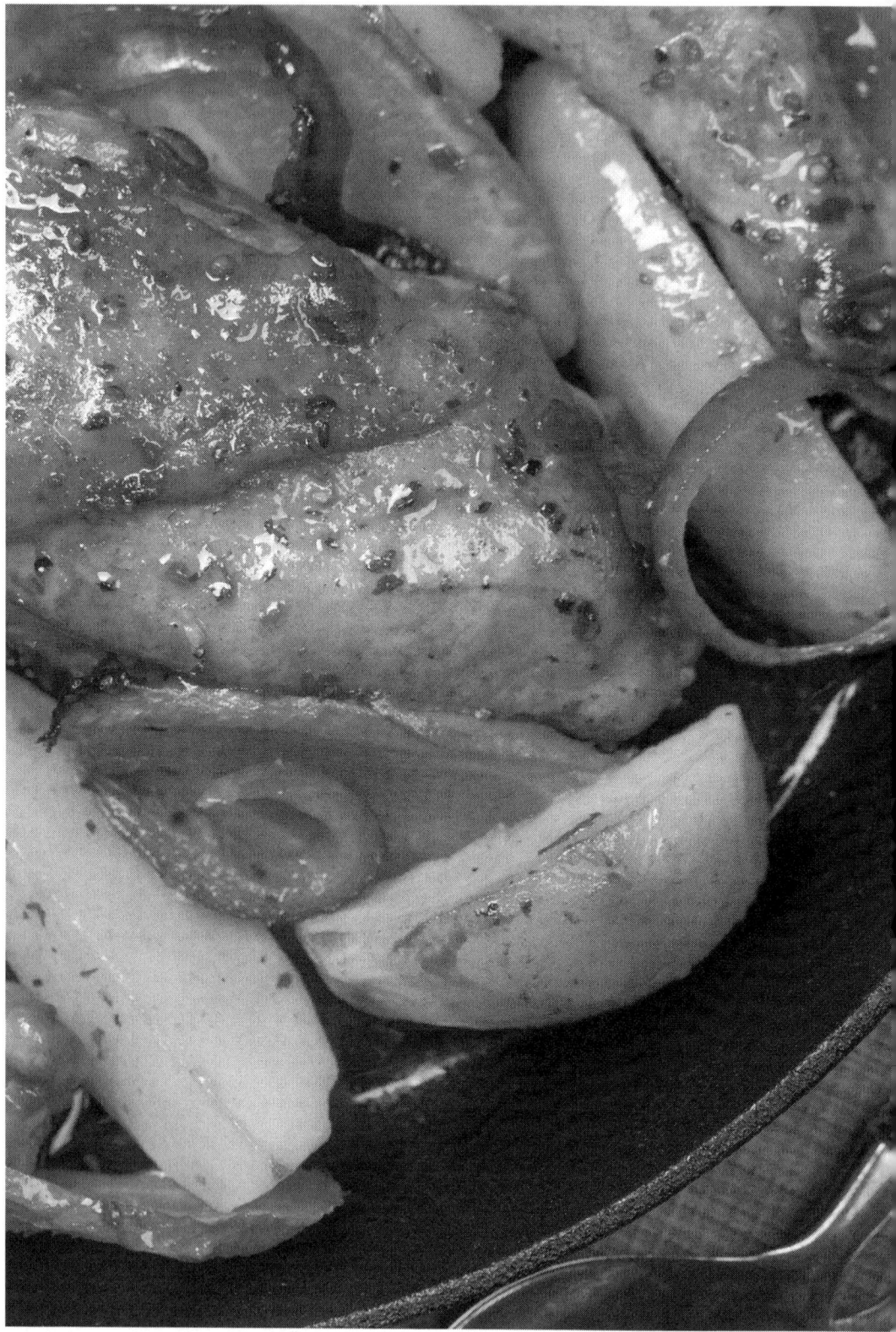

Chapter 11

Keto Diet Recipes

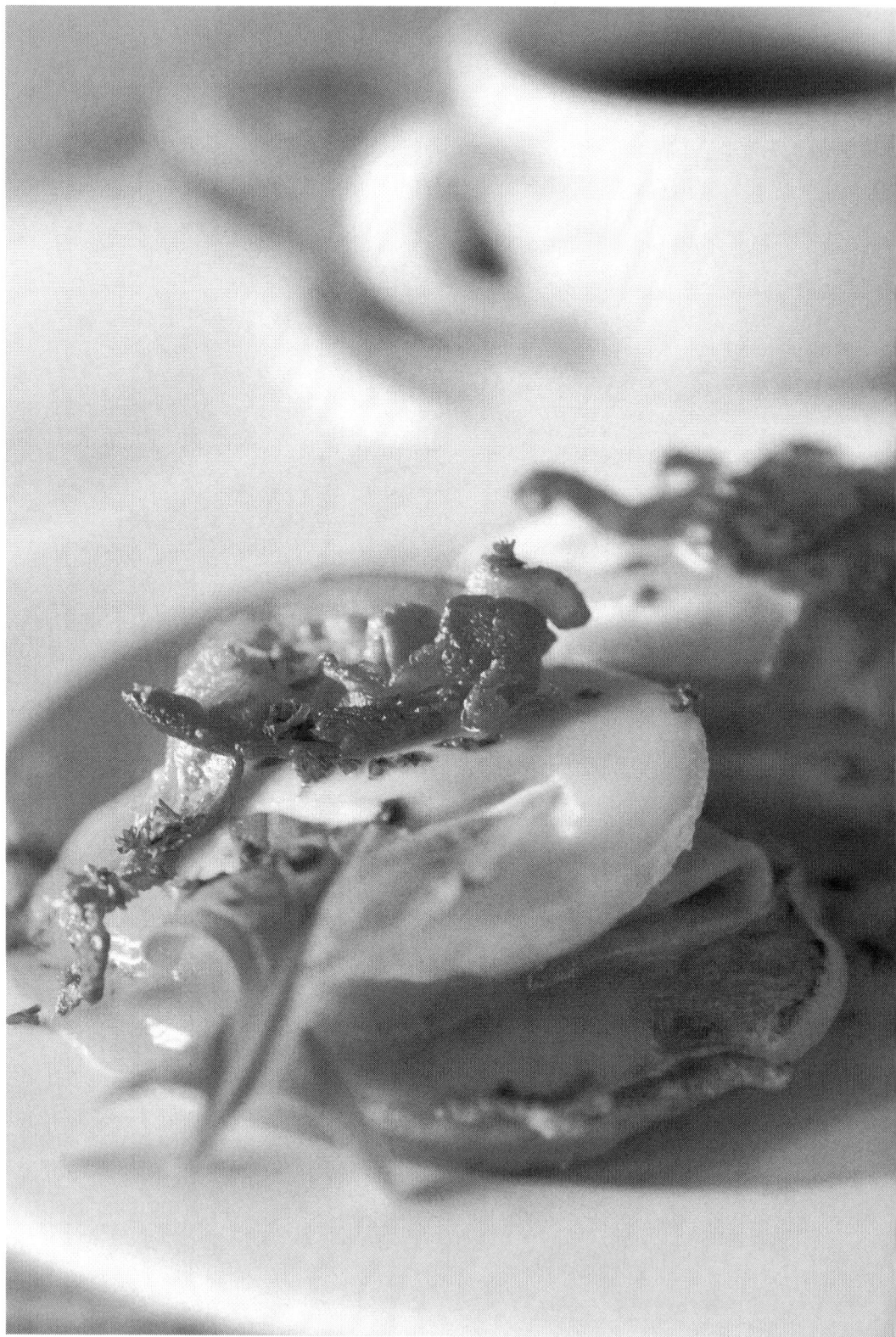

One Pan Breakfast

I don't know about you, but my day will surely be a lot better when I have bacon and eggs for breakfast. I mean, how can you go wrong with this combo?

Here's my one-pan breakfast recipe with bacon and eggs.

Portion

This recipe is for 3-4 persons.

Total Time

30 mins.

Ingredients

- 8 slices bacon
- 4 pcs. free-range eggs
- 1 medium-sized carrots julienned
- ½ cup celery, chopped
- ½ cup cauliflower, chopped
- 1 small white onion, chopped
- ½ cup gouda cheese, shredded
- 1 tbsp. butter

Nutritional Values

- ✓ Calories: 385 kcal
- ✓ Fat: 33.05g (66%)
- ✓ Carbohydrates: 5.58g (4%)

✓ Protein: 16.19g (30%)
✓ Dietary Fiber: 1.2g
✓ Cholesterol: 629mg

How to Make the Dish

➢ Prepare the vegetables and bacon.
➢ Heat a large pan over medium fire and add the 1 tbsp. butter to melt.
➢ Throw in the chopped vegetables and bacon and sauté for 20 mins or until the bacon is almost crisp. Remember to stir often.
➢ Using a spatula, spread the vegetables and bacon evenly on the pan and then create four well.
➢ Take one egg and then break it into the well. Do the same for the rest of the eggs.
➢ Cover the pan with a lid and then heat until the eggs are cooked to your liking.
➢ Turn off the heat and then sprinkle with the shredded cheese. Serve.

All-in Omelet

This is a level-up recipe for the classic breakfast food. Delicious and easy to make!

Portion

This recipe is good for 2 persons.

Total Time

10 mins.

Ingredients

- 4 eggs whites from a free range egg
- 1 pc. yolk
- 1 pc. heirloom tomato, chopped
- 1 cup baby spinach, roughly chopped
- ¼ cup cheddar, shredded
- 1 small white onion, chopped
- ½ tsp. dried basil
- 2 tbsp. coconut milk
- 1 tbsp. butter

Nutritional Values

- ✓ Calories: 601 kcal
- ✓ Fat: 33.57g (68%)
- ✓ Carbohydrates: 8.95g (8%)
- ✓ Protein: 25.29g (24%)
- ✓ Dietary Fiber : 1.5g
- ✓ Cholesterol: 1363mg

How to Make the Dish

- ➢ Place all the egg whites and yolk in a mixing bowl. Add the 2 tbsp. coconut milk and whisk all the ingredients together.
- ➢ Melt the butter on a non-stick pan over medium fire. Throw in the baby spinach, cheddar, chopped tomato, and onion. Sauté for 5 minutes or until the spinach is wilted. Set aside.
- ➢ Transfer the sautéed vegetables on a plate and set aside.
- ➢ Pour the egg mixture into the same pan and cook the eggs until done.
- ➢ Place the cooked egg on a serving plate and then top one half of the egg with the cooked vegetables. Fold the egg and to create an omelet. Serve.

Heavenly Cups

This recipe is a personal favorite. I love it because it's a no-brainer to cook and prepare, plus it's as convenient as a breakfast to-go.

Portion

This recipe is for 3 persons.

Total Time

25 mins.

Ingredients

- 6 free-range eggs
- 350 grams ham, cooked and cut into cubes
- 1 yellow onion, chopped
- 2 tbsp. onion chopped chives
- 1 cup shredded cheddar
- 3 tbsp. plus 1 tbsp. butter
- ½ cup heavy cream

Nutritional Values

- ✓ Calories: 420 kcal
- ✓ Fat: 31.87g (68%)
- ✓ Carbohydrates: 7.55g (7%)
- ✓ Protein: 25.52g (26%)
- ✓ Dietary Fiber : 0.7g
- ✓ Cholesterol: 1291mg

How to Make the Dish

- ➢ Preheat the oven at 400F.
- ➢ Melt the 3 tbsp. butter in a skillet heated over medium fire.
- ➢ Add the onions to the pan and sauté until the onions are translucent. Add the garlic and sauté for another minute or two. Turn off the heat and transfer the in a large bowl.
- ➢ Add the rest of the ingredients in the bowl with the sautéed vegetables except for the 1 tbsp. butter. Stir well and set aside.
- ➢ Take 6 pcs. of ramekins and brush it with the 1 tbsp. butter. Pour the mixture into the prepared ramekins filling only ½ of the cups.
- ➢ Place in the oven to cook for 20 minutes or until the top turns light brown. Serve.

Pesto and Eggs

Are you a fan of pesto? Then you'll surely love this breakfast recipe! It's delicious and can give you the energy boost you'll need in the morning.

Portion

This recipe is good for 2 persons.

Total Time

10 mins.

Ingredients

- 1 ½ tbsp. pesto sauce
- 4 free-range eggs
- 2 tbsp. butter
- 3 tbsp. source cream

Nutritional Values

- ✓ Calories: 210 kcal
- ✓ Fat: 22.46g (94%)
- ✓ Carbohydrates: 1.31g (3%)
- ✓ Protein: 1.9g (3%)
- ✓ Dietary Fiber : 0.1g
- ✓ Cholesterol: 47mg

How to Make the Dish

- ➢ Whisk the eggs in a bowl. You can lightly season it with salt and pepper.
- ➢ Heat a non-stick pan over medium fire. Melt the butter and then pour the whisked egg on the hot pan.
- ➢ Add the pesto sauce to the pan and stir.
- ➢ Turn off the heat and then add the 3 scoops of sour cream. Stir well.
- ➢ You can serve with on the side of a mashed avocado.

Ketogenic Pancakes

Besides eggs and bacon, another breakfast comfort food that tops my list (and probably your list also) are pancakes. Good thing, there is a ketogenic diet friendly recipe for pancakes. You should really try this one!

Portion

This recipe is for a family of 5.

Total Time

20 mins.

Ingredients

- 4 large free-range eggs
- ¾ cup nut butter
- ½ tsp. baking soda
- 1 tsp. cinnamon powder
- 1/3 cup coconut milk
- 2 tbsp. of a sugar substitute like stevia or erythritol
- 2 tbsp. butter or clarified butter

Nutritional Values

- ✓ Calories: 329 kcal
- ✓ Fat: 29.11g (75%)
- ✓ Carbohydrates: 13.32g (16%)
- ✓ Protein: 7.39g (8%)
- ✓ Dietary Fiber : 1.4g
- ✓ Cholesterol: 161mg

How to Make the Dish

- ➢ Add all the ingredients in a food processor (except the 2 tbsp. butter) and pulse until all the ingredients are thoroughly combined. Set aside.
- ➢ Melt the butter on a non-stick pan over low fire. Scoop ¼ cup of the pancake batter into the hot pan and then cook until the pancake has set, flip and cook until finished.
- ➢ Repeat the same procedure for the rest of the batter. You can serve this with a drizzle of an all-natural maple syrup.

Bread-Free Sandwich

Of course you need to cut down on bread when you're on a low-carb diet. Since I couldn't skip not eating sandwich, I made one that didn't use bread and was successful at it!

Portion

This recipe is for 2 persons.

Total Time

15 mins.

Ingredients

- 4 large free-range eggs
- 2 slices of pre-cooked ham
- 4 tbsp. provolone cheese, cut into thick slices
- A dash of Sriracha sauce
- A pinch of salt and pepper to taste
- 1 tbsp. butter

Nutritional Values

- ✓ Calories: 253 kcal
- ✓ Fat: 17.96g (63%)
- ✓ Carbohydrates: 6.9g (10%)
- ✓ Protein: 15.99g (26%)
- ✓ Dietary Fiber : 0.3g
- ✓ Cholesterol: 399mg

How to Make the Dish

- ➢ Melt the butter on a non-stick pan over medium fire. Crack the eggs, season with salt and pepper and fry until over easy.
- ➢ Sandwich the slices of ham and cheese in between 2 cooked eggs.
- ➢ Add a dash of Sriracha for an added kick (optional) and serve.

Cheesy Sausage Pie

Here is a recipe of a delicious breakfast pie that you can make ahead and warm in the oven for breakfast.

Portion

This recipe makes 2 ramekin size pie.

Total Time

35 mins.

Ingredients

- ¾ cup plus 2 tbsp. cheddar cheese, grated
- 2 pcs. chicken sausages
- ¼ cup coconut flour
- ¼ tsp. baking soda
- ½ tsp rosemary
- ¼ tsp. cayenne
- A pinch of kosher salt
- 5 egg yolks (free range)
- ¼ cup coconut oil
- 2 tbsp. coconut milk
- 2 tsp. lime juice

Nutritional Values

- ✓ Calories: 613 kcal
- ✓ Fat: 55.06g (79%)
- ✓ Carbohydrates: 5.39g (3%)
- ✓ Protein: 24.84g (18%)
- ✓ Dietary Fiber : 0.4g
- ✓ Cholesterol: 1562mg

How to Make the Dish

- ➢ Preheat oven at 350F.
- ➢ Slice the chicken sausages into small chunks and place on a heated skillet greased with butter.
- ➢ While waiting for the sausages to cook, combine the ¼ cup cheddar, coconut flour, baking soda, rosemary, cayenne, and salt in a mixing bowl.
- ➢ In a separate bowl, mix the yolks, coconut oil, coconut milk, and lime juice. Stir well.
- ➢ Gradually add the wet ingredients into the bowl with the dry ingredients and fold to incorporate all the ingredients together.
- ➢ Pour the mixture into 2 ramekins and add the cooked sausages also in the ramekins.
- ➢ Place in the oven to cook for 25 minutes or until the pies turn light brown.
- ➢ Add the remaining cheddar on top of the pies and place back in the oven to melt the cheese for 4-5 minutes. Serve.

Egg and Avocado Salad

Don't worry if you're not yet too confident with your skills in the kitchen. You will surely ace this simple breakfast salad recipe.

Portion

This salad recipe is good for 2-3 persons.

Total Time

15 mins.

Ingredients

- 4 pcs. free range eggs
- 1 oc. avocado
- 1 tsp. Dijon mustard
- ¼ cup mayonnaise
- 2 tbsp. cream cheese
- 1 scallion, chopped
- A pinch of kosher salt and pepper to taste

Nutritional Values

- ✓ Calories: 382 kcal
- ✓ Fat: 31.99g (74%)
- ✓ Carbohydrates: 9.91g (9%)
- ✓ Protein: 16.65g (17%)
- ✓ Dietary Fiber : 5.1g
- ✓ Cholesterol: 834mg

How to Make the Dish

➢ Boil the eggs in a pot for 10 mins. When done, run the boiled eggs with tap water. Remove the peel and then chop.

➢ In a mixing bowl, combine the chopped eggs, mustard, mayo, cream cheese, and scallion. Lightly season it salt and pepper.

➢ Cut the avocado in half and scoop out the flesh. Discard the peel and pit and add the flesh into the egg salad. Serve.

Full-Plate Breakfast

There are times when you're just too lazy to cook for breakfast, but that's no excuse to not eating a healthy keto-friendly plate. This recipe is very easy and fast to prepare, giving you no excuse not to make breakfast.

Portion

This recipe is for one person with a big appetite.

Total Time

10 mins.

Ingredients

- 2 cups Portobello mushrooms, chopped
- 5 bacon strips
- 1 small ripe avocado, chopped
- 1 free-range egg
- A pinch of salt and pepper to taste

Nutritional Values

- ✓ Calories: 441 kcal
- ✓ Fat: 37.5g (71%)
- ✓ Carbohydrates: 24.98g (20%)
- ✓ Protein: 12.62g (9%)
- ✓ Dietary Fiber : 16g
- ✓ Cholesterol: 0mg

How to Make the Dish

> - Heat a skillet and then cook the bacon.
> - When done, place the bacon strips on a plate and use the fat to cook the mushrooms.
> - Sauté the mushrooms in the bacon fat for 5 minutes. Lightly season with salt and pepper.
> - Remove the mushrooms from the pan and the cook the egg (sunny side up)
> - Serve the bacon strips, mushrooms, egg, and chopped avocado on a single plate and devour!

Keto-Friendly Porridge

High in fat, low in carbs, this recipe is a perfect ketogenic diet porridge.

Portion

This recipe is for 2 bowls of coco porridge goodness.

Total Time

10 mins.

Ingredients

- 2 free-range eggs
- 2 tbsp. coconut flour
- 8 tbsp. coconut cream
- ¼ tsp. psyllium husk powder, ground
- ¼ tsp salt
- 4 tbsp. butter

Nutritional Values

- ✓ Calories: 415 kcal
- ✓ Fat: 34.39g (73%)
- ✓ Carbohydrates: 15.7g (15%)
- ✓ Protein: 11.45g (12%)
- ✓ Dietary Fiber : 0.2g
- ✓ Cholesterol: 684mg

How to Make the Dish

- ➢ Place all the ingredients on a saucepan over low-heat.
- ➢ Stir consistently and cook for 10 minutes, or until you achieve your desired consistency.

Serve with a splash of coconut milk with some pieces of berries on top.

Roasted Veg and Egg

This is a recipe I discovered by accident. It was a weekend and I haven't gone the grocery yet to re-fill my food stock. So what I did was to take whatever I had left and made it into this awesome dish.

Portion

This recipe is for 1 person.

Total Time

35 mins.

Ingredients

- 2 cups cauliflower florets, chopped
- 1 cup broccoli florets, chopped
- 1 free-range egg
- ½ tsp. red pepper flakes
- ¼ tsp. garlic powder
- A pinch of salt and pepper
- ¼ tsp. paprika
- ½ lemon, juiced
- 2 tbsp. olive oil
- 1 tbsp. butter
- A dash of Sriracha sauce (optional)

Nutritional Values

- ✓ Calories: 349 kcal
- ✓ Fat: 19.49g (64%)

- ✓ Carbohydrates: 13.28g (17%)
- ✓ Protein: 14.59g (19%)
- ✓ Dietary Fiber : 5.2g

How to Make the Dish

➢ Set the oven at 400F.
➢ Place the veggies in a large bowl. Season with the red pepper flakes, garlic powder, salt, and pepper. Drizzle the olive oil and toss the veggies.
➢ Transfer the veggies on a baking sheet lined with foil. Drizzle with the lemon juice on top and place in the oven to roast for 15 minutes.
➢ Toss the veggies halfway through roasting.
➢ When the veggies are almost one cooking in the oven, prepare the egg by melting the butter on a nonstick pan heated over medium fire. Crack the egg and season with the paprika, salt, and pepper. Set aside.
➢ Place the roasted veggies on a serving plate and add the egg on top. Add a dash of Sriracha and enjoy.

CHICKEN RECIPES

Roasted Chicken Thighs

This recipe is ideal to make for the weekends as it takes time to bake the chicken and allow the juices to ooze out from the tender meat. Nevertheless, it's a meal worth waiting for!

Portion

This recipe is for a group of 5.

Total Time

2 hrs. 15 mins.

Ingredients

- 2 lbs. boneless chicken thighs
- 1 tbsp. garlic granules
- 2 tbsp. garlic flakes
- 1 tbsp. chopped parsley
- 2 tbsp. coconut aminos
- 1 tsp. melted butter
- Kosher salt and pepper to taste

Nutritional Values

- ✓ Calories: 420 kcal
- ✓ Fat: 30.96g (66%)
- ✓ Carbohydrates: 3.26g (3%)
- ✓ Protein: 30.55g (31%)
- ✓ Dietary Fiber : 0.3g

✓ Cholesterol: 180mg

How to Make the Dish

- ➢ Preheat the oven at 300F.
- ➢ Place 2 layers of foil on a baking sheet and arrange the boneless chicken thighs on top.
- ➢ Season with thighs with the garlic, onion, salt and pepper.
- ➢ Wrap the chicken with foil making sure it is well sealed.
- ➢ Place in the oven to roast for 2 hours.
- ➢ When done, open the foil and transfer the drippings in a bowl and set aside.
- ➢ Allow the chicken to cool for a bit before slicing it into bite-sized pieces.
- ➢ Place the chicken chunks in a serving platter along with the flavorful juices. Serve warm.

Baked Chicken in Creamy Herb Sauce

Delicious and indulgent—these are the two words that best describe this recipe. This is the dish I go to when I impress my loved ones; and it has never failed me!

Portion

This recipe is good for 4 persons.

Total Time

55 mins.

Ingredients

- 4 pcs. boneless chicken breast
- 5 tbsp. butter (divided into 2 2 tbsps., 1 tbsp.)
- 3 cloves of garlic
- 1 medium sized onion, sliced thin
- 1 ½ Herbes de Provence
- 1 tsp. tarragon
- A pinch of kosher salt to taste
- 1 cup cream cheese
- ½ cup heavy cream
- ½ cup chicken broth
- ½ cup dry white wine

Nutritional Values

- ✓ Calories: 704 kcal
- ✓ Fat: 51.12g (66%)

- ✓ Carbohydrates: 3.94g (2%)
- ✓ Protein: 53.89g (32%)
- ✓ Dietary Fiber : 0.1g
- ✓ Cholesterol: 251mg

How to Make the Dish

- ➢ Preheat oven at 350F.
- ➢ Place a pan over medium fire and melt 2 tbsp. of butter. Add the garlic, onion and tarragon and sauté for 2-3 minutes. Set aside when done.
- ➢ Place the same pan over low heat and melt another 2 tbsp. of butter. Add the dry white wine and cream cheese. Stir until the cream cheese is melted. Add the heavy cream to the pan along with salt and Herbes de Provence. Stir well and set aside.
- ➢ Meanwhile, grease a baking pan with the remaining 1 tbsp. of butter. Pour the chicken broth in the pan and then the chicken breasts.
- ➢ Serve with green salad on the side.
- ➢ Take the sautéed garlic and onion as well as the prepared sauce and spoon on top of the chicken.
- ➢ Place in the oven to bake for 45 mins.

Homemade Chicken Nuggets

Skip the unhealthy and processed store-bought nuggets and make one at home. Here's my recipe of a garlicky chicken nuggets.

Portion

This recipe is for 2 persons.

Total Time

25 mins.

Ingredients

- 2 pcs. boneless chicken thighs, cut into cubes
- ½ cup coconut flour
- 1 tsp. kosher salt
- 2 tbsp. garlic powder
- 1 free-range egg
- ½ cup clarified butter or ghee

Nutritional Values

- ✓ Calories: 959 kcal
- ✓ Fat: 80.9g (75%)
- ✓ Carbohydrates: 28.75g (12%)
- ✓ Protein: 31.82g (13%)
- ✓ Dietary Fiber : 1.5g
- ✓ Cholesterol: 547mg

How to Make the Dish

- ➢ In a bowl combine the coconut flour, salt, and garlic powder. You can adjust the flavor per your liking.
- ➢ Whisk the egg in another bowl.
- ➢ Heat the clarified butter in a saucepan over medium fire.
- ➢ Dip the chicken cubes in the egg and then into the flour mixture.
- ➢ Place the chicken cubes one by one in the saucepan to fry the nuggets. This may take approximately 10 minutes to get a perfect golden brown.
- ➢ Serve.

Hearty Chicken Soup

Whether it's cold outside or I'm feeling a little bit under the weather, this is a dish I'd love to prepare. Take note though, that you need a crockpot for this one and will also have to wait 6 hours to get a taste of the delicious hearty soup.

Portion

This recipe is good for sharing among 5 people.

Total Time

6 hrs. and 15 mins.

Ingredients

- 3 pcs. boneless chicken thighs
- ¼ cup Sriracha sauce
- 3 cups low-sodium beef broth
- ¼ cup butter
- 1 tsp. onion powder
- 1 tsp. garlic powder
- ¼ tsp. celery seeds
- 1 cup heavy cream
- ½ cup cream cheese
- ¼ tsp. Xanthan gum
- A pinch of kosher salt and pepper to taste

Nutritional Values

- ✓ Calories: 617 kcal
- ✓ Fat: 42.41g (66%)

✓ Carbohydrates: 29.9g (16%)
✓ Protein: 24.21g (15%)
✓ Dietary Fiber : 0.8g
✓ Cholesterol: 147mg

How to Make the Dish

➢ Place in chicken cubes first in the crock pot and then followed by the rest of the ingredients except the cream cheese, heavy cream, and Xanthan gum.
➢ Slow cook on low for 6 hours.
➢ When done, remove the chicken and shred using a fork.
➢ Add the rest of the ingredients into the crockpot and use an immersion blender to combine all the ingredients together.
➢ Place the shredded chicken back into the pot and season with salt and pepper. Serve hot.

Chicken Meatballs

I experienced a phase where I just can't get enough of meatballs, that's why I tried a number of recipes made of different meats and this recipe tops my list as one of my favorites.

Portion

This recipe is for 2 persons.

Total Time

30 mins.

Ingredients

- ½ lb. chicken thigh, ground
- ¾ cup cheddar, shredded
- 2 tbsp. almond flour
- 2 tbsp. flaxseed meal
- 2 tbsp. fresh cilantro, chopped
- 2 pcs. scallions, chopped
- 1 small bell pepper, chopped
- ½ tsp. garlic powder
- ¼ tsp. red pepper flakes
- A pinch of kosher salt and pepper to taste
- 1 juice of lemon
- 1 tsp. lemon zest

Nutritional Values

- ✓ Calories: 547 kcal
- ✓ Fat: 40.72g (66%)

- ✓ Carbohydrates: 12.52g (8%)
- ✓ Protein: 34.31g (25%)
- ✓ Dietary Fiber : 4.3g
- ✓ Cholesterol: 162mg

How to Make the Dish

- ➢ Preheat oven at 350F.
- ➢ In a large bowl, combine all the ingredients together. Use your hands to make sure that everything is well incorporated.
- ➢ Shape the mixture into balls of about 2 inches in diameter.
- ➢ Line a baking sheet with foil and place the chicken balls on top.
- ➢ Place in the oven to bake for 20 minutes.
- ➢ You can serve these meatballs with mashed avocado on the side.

Chicken and Parmesan Patties

Meaty and cheesy goodness on your plate, that's one delicious dish. Do you agree?

Portion

This recipe is for 1-2 persons.

Total Time

30 mins.

Ingredients

- 2 pcs. boneless chicken thighs
- ¼ cup parmesan cheese
- 4 pcs. bacon strips
- 1 free-range egg
- 1 large bell pepper, sliced
- ¼ cup tomato paste
- 3 tbsp. almond flour

Nutritional Values

- ✓ Calories: 630 kcal
- ✓ Fat: 41.21g (59%)
- ✓ Carbohydrates: 30.56g (12%)
- ✓ Protein: 41.21g (22%)
- ✓ Dietary Fiber : 2.2g
- ✓ Cholesterol: 436mg

How to Make the Dish

- ➢ Boil the chicken and then cut into chunks. You can cook the bacon while boiling the chicken.
- ➢ Using a food processor, finely chop the bell pepper. When done drain the excess liquid and transfer the chopped peppers into a bowl.
- ➢ When your meat is cooked place the chicken with the bacon strips in the food processor and pulse until you achieve a smooth consistency.
- ➢ Add the meat into the bowl with the bell pepper. Also add the tomato paste, parmesan cheese, egg and almond flour. Combine well using your hands.
- ➢ Create patties with the mixture of an about 3 inches in diameter.
- ➢ Grease a pan with butter and heat over medium fire. Cook each side of the patty until light brown and crisp. Serve.

Chicken Filled Zucchini Boats

Once in a while I have my friends over at my house and would want to serve delicious ketogenic dishes for them. One of my go-to recipes is this chicken filled zucchini dish that are a usual hit with my guests.

Portion

This recipe serves a party of 4.

Total Time

40 mins.

Ingredients

- 4 pcs. medium-sized zucchini
- 1 ½ cup rotisserie chicken, shredded
- 2 cups broccoli florets
- ¼ cup cheddar, shredded
- 2 tbsp. sour cream
- 4 tbsp. butter, melted
- 1 tbsp. onion chive, chopped
- A pinch of salt and pepper to taste

Nutritional Values

- ✓ Calories: 491 kcal
- ✓ Fat: 29.84g (54%)
- ✓ Carbohydrates: 2.73g (2%)
- ✓ Protein: 54.13g (44%)
- ✓ Dietary Fiber : 0.8g
- ✓ Cholesterol: 214mg

How to Make the Dish

- ➢ Preheat oven at 400F.
- ➢ Cut the zucchini into half (lengthwise) and then remove the insides with the spoon.
- ➢ Pour the melted butter into the zucchini boats and then lightly season with salt and pepper.
- ➢ Place in the oven to bake for 20 minutes.
- ➢ While waiting for the zucchini boats, chop the broccoli florets and transfer into a mixing bowl. Add the shredded chicken, cheddar, sour cream and mix well.
- ➢ When the boats are done, take it out from the oven and fill the boats with the chicken and cheese mixture.
- ➢ Place back in the oven to bake for another 15 minutes. Garnish with the chopped chives before serving.

Parmesan Dusted Wings

Along with the zucchini boats, this is another dish I like serving when I have guests coming over to my house.

Portion

This recipe serves a party of 4.

Total Time

40 mins.

Ingredients

- 20 pcs. chicken wings
- 1 cup parmesan cheese, grated
- 2 tsp. dried oregano
- A pinch of salt to taste
- ½ tbsp. garlic powder
- 2 tbsp. butter

Nutritional Values

- ✓ Calories: 344 kcal
- ✓ Fat: 17.88g (46%)
- ✓ Carbohydrates: 4.72g (5%)
- ✓ Protein: 39.27g (49%)
- ✓ Dietary Fiber : 0.3g
- ✓ Cholesterol: 119mg

How to Make the Dish

- ➤ Set oven at 450F.
- ➤ Grease a baking pan with 2 tbsp. of butter and place the chicken wings in it.
- ➤ Season with the dried oregano and salt and place in the oven to bake for 35 minutes or until done.
- ➤ When cooked, remove the chicken wings from the oven and place on a large bowl. Sprinkle the wings with the grated parmesan and garlic powder.
- ➤ Shake until the wings are well coated. Serve.

Chicken Tenderloins Done Right

Chicken tenderloins are the short and thin cuts taken from underneath the chicken breast. This recipe is a casserole dish made with chicken tenderloins and prosciutto.

Portion

This recipe is good for a group of 6.

Total Time

15 mins.

Ingredients

- 2 lbs. chicken tenderloins
- 115g prosciutto, chopped
- 1 ½ cup Brussels sprouts
- ½ cup low-sodium chicken broth
- 1 ½ cup heavy cream
- 1 pc. lemon juiced
- 2 cloves of garlic minced
- Clarified butter for frying

Nutritional Values

- ✓ Calories: 463 kcal
- ✓ Fat: 32.86 (63%)
- ✓ Carbohydrates: 3.94g (3%)
- ✓ Protein: 37.66g (34%)
- ✓ Dietary Fiber : 0.9g
- ✓ Cholesterol: 196mg

How to Make the Dish

- ➢ Set the oven at 400F.
- ➢ Cut the Brussels sprouts in half and then place in a pot with boiling water. Cook for 5 minutes and set aside when done.
- ➢ Meanwhile heat the broth in a saucepan on medium fire and bring into a boil.
- ➢ When boiling, add the heavy cream, lemon juice and minced garlic into the pot and allow to simmer for 10 minutes. Remember to stir frequently. Turn off heat when done and set aside.
- ➢ In another pan, heat the clarified butter on medium-high fire. When hot, add the chicken tenderloins and then the chopped prosciutto when the chicken is almost done.
- ➢ Take a casserole dish and add the cooked Brussels sprouts at the bottom followed by the chicken and prosciutto, and finally, the garlic-lemon cream.
- ➢ Bake in the oven to for 20 minutes. Serve.

Slow-Cooked Spicy Chicken

I always believe that food that is cooked slowly is always a winner—and this recipe proves that I'm right. Preparing this dish is easy as it is cooking it. You just need to let your crockpot do its magic!

Portion

This recipe is for 4 people.

Total Time

7 hours and 5 mins.

Ingredients

- 6 pcs. chicken breast, frozen
- ¼ cup cayenne pepper sauce
- 3/4 cup ranch sauce
- 4 tbsp. butter

Nutritional Values

- ✓ Calories: 869 kcal
- ✓ Fat: 51.87g (53%)
- ✓ Carbohydrates: 4.38g (2%)
- ✓ Protein: 91.82g (45%)
- ✓ Dietary Fiber : 1.2g
- ✓ Cholesterol: 309mg

How to Make the Dish

- ➢ Add the chicken at the bottom of the slow cooker. Pour the cayenne pepper sauce and ranch sauce on top. Stir gently to make sure the chicken is coated with the sauce.
- ➢ Cover the pot and cook on low for 6 hours.
- ➢ Remove the cover after 6 hours and then add the butter on top.
- ➢ Cook again for another hour on low, without the lid on top.
- ➢ Serve.

BEEF RECIPES

Slow-Cooked Herbed Beef

Have I told you yet? I love slow-cooked dishes. Not only because they're delicious, but also they're easy to make. Just prepare the ingredients place in your crockpot to cook for a few hours, *voila!* You have a mouthwatering dish!

Portion

This recipe is for a group of 4.

Total Time

8 hours and 10 mins.

Ingredients

- 1 ½ lbs. beef tenderloin, sliced
- 2 pcs. celery, chopped
- 1 cup low-sodium beef broth
- 2 tsp. dried thyme
- 2 tsp. dried marjoram
- 1 tsp. Dijon mustard
- A pinch of salt and pepper
- 2 tbsp. butter
- 2 tbsp. amaranth flour
- 2 tbsp. olive oil
- 4 tbsp. parsley, chopped
- 2 tbsp. freshly squeezed lemon juice

Nutritional Values

- ✓ Calories: 531 kcal
- ✓ Fat: 29.34g (49%)
- ✓ Carbohydrates: 9.73g (7%)
- ✓ Protein: 55.48g (44%)
- ✓ Dietary Fiber : 1.5g
- ✓ Cholesterol: 177mg

How to Make the Dish

- ➢ Dust the tenderloin with the flour.
- ➢ Melt the butter on a skillet over medium fire and then add the beef and cook until brown.
- ➢ Transfer the beef into the slow cooker and then add the rest of the ingredients into the pot except the parsley and lemon juice.
- ➢ Cover the pot and cook slowly on low for 8 hours.
- ➢ When done, drizzle the lemon juice and sprinkle with parsley on top. Stir well and serve.

Beefy Tacos

This is a classic taco recipe with a healthier twist.

Portion

This recipe is for a group of 5 people.

Total Time

25 mins.

Ingredients

- 1 lb. ground beef
- 2 tbsp. butter
- 3 cloves of garlic, minced
- 1 small onion, chopped
- 1 small can of green chilies
- 1 tsp. coriander, ground
- 2 tsp. chili powder
- ½ cups sour cream
- 2 cups cheddar cheese, grated
- Lettuce cups for the wrap

Nutritional Values

- ✓ Calories: 475 kcal
- ✓ Fat: 29.97g (57%)
- ✓ Carbohydrates: 14.22g (12%)
- ✓ Protein: 36.47g (32%)
- ✓ Dietary Fiber : 0.8g
- ✓ Cholesterol: 135mg

How to Make the Dish

- ➢ Melt the butter in a pan over medium fire and then sauté the onion and garlic until soft.
- ➢ Add the ground beef and then cook until done.
- ➢ Add the green chilies, coriander and chili powder. Mix well and allow to cook for 5 minutes.
- ➢ Turn the heat to low and then add the sour cream and cheddar. Cook for another 15 minutes.
- ➢ Scoop the prepared taco filling into lettuce cups and serve.

Beef Stir-Fry

Want to have a taste of Asian dish for your meals? This is the one you should try! My Korean friend who's also into the Keto diet shared this recipe to me, so I'm sharing it to you too. Enjoy!

Portion

This recipe is good for 5 people.

Total Time

20 mins.

Ingredients

- 1 ¼ lb. ground beef
- 1 tbsp. clarified butter
- 3 cloves of garlic
- ¼ tsp. ginger, minced
- 1 tsp. red pepper flakes
- ¼ cup coconut aminos
- ½ tsp. liquid stevia
- ½ tsp. molasses
- 2 pcs. green onions, chopped

Nutritional Values

- ✓ Calories: 324 kcal
- ✓ Fat: 20.93g (58%)
- ✓ Carbohydrates: 3.28g (4%)
- ✓ Protein: 29.15g (38%)
- ✓ Dietary Fiber : 0.7g
- ✓ Cholesterol: 106mg

How to Make the Dish

- ➢ Place a wok or skillet over medium fire. Melt the butter and then add the ground beef. Cook for a few minutes until brown.
- ➢ Add the liquid stevia, coconut aminos, molasses and red pepper flakes and then stir and allow to simmer for 3-4 minutes.
- ➢ Garnish with chopped green onions on top before serving.

Beef Balls in Creamy Sauce

This recipe is a bombshell of flavors. I couldn't get enough of this dish the first time I ate it. You should try it too!

Portion

This recipe is good for 4 people.

Total Time

30 mins.

Ingredients

- 1 ½ lb. ground beef
- 2 tbsp. Worcestershire sauce
- 3 tbsp. fresh parsley, chopped
- 3 cloves of garlic, minced
- 1 tsp. garlic powder
- 1 small onion, diced
- 1 tsp. onion powder
- Salt and pepper to taste
- 2 tbsp. clarified butter
- 2 tbsp. butter
- ½ cup sliced button mushrooms
- 1 cup low-sodium beef stock
- 2 tbsp. cooking sherry
- 2 tbsp. beef bouillon granules
- ¼ cup heavy cream
- ¾ cup sour cream

Nutritional Values

- ✓ Calories: 714 kcal
- ✓ Fat: 48.49g (60%)
- ✓ Carbohydrates: 19.73g (11%)
- ✓ Protein: 49.25g (29%)
- ✓ Dietary Fiber : 1.1g
- ✓ Cholesterol: 210mg

How to Make the Dish

➢ In a large bowl, mix together the ground beef, one clove of the minced garlic, chopped parsley, Worcestershire, garlic powder and onion powder. Season with salt and pepper. Combine the ingredients with your hands and then create 4 patties.

➢ Heat the clarified butter in a pan over medium-high fire. Place the patties and sear for about 2 minutes on each side. Remove the patties and set aside.

➢ Using the same pan, melt the butter and drizzle the cooking sherry. Lower the fire and add the diced onion, button mushrooms, and the rest of the minced garlic. Cook until the onions are caramelized.

➢ Pour the beef stock into the pan and also add the bouillon granules.

➢ Add the heavy cream and sour cream into the pan, followed by the browned patties. Allow to simmer on low fire for 10 minutes. Serve.

Beefy, Gooey Cheese, Goodness

The name says it all! This I a quick recipe to make that will surely be a hit with those who love cheese.

Portion

This recipe is good for sharing between 4 people.

Total Time

55 mins.

Ingredients

- 1 lb. ground beef
- 1 cup cheddar cheese, grated
- 1 cup baby spinach, chopped
- 1 small bell pepper, chopped
- 5 free-range eggs
- A dash of salt and pepper to taste

Nutritional Values

- ✓ Calories: 391 kcal
- ✓ Fat: 22.41g (51%)
- ✓ Carbohydrates: 7.61g (7%)
- ✓ Protein: 40.85g (41%)
- ✓ Dietary Fiber : 1.4g
- ✓ Cholesterol: 333mg

How to Make the Dish

- ➢ Set the oven at 350F.
- ➢ Place the ground beef on a skillet and cook until brown.
- ➢ Transfer the cooked beef on a mixing bowl and then add the baby spinach and red pepper. Combine well.
- ➢ Place the beef and spinach mixture into a baking dish greased with butter making sure it is well distributed onto the dish.
- ➢ On another bowl, whisk the eggs and season with salt and pepper.
- ➢ Add the cheddar cheese on top of the beef and then followed by the whisked egg.
- ➢ Place the in the oven to bake for 18-20 minutes. Allow to cool for a few minutes before cutting into squares and serving.

Beef Sausage and Bacon Pot

This recipe looks like a breakfast meal, but I surely love eating this even for lunch or dinner. You decide when you want to have it best!

Portion

This recipe is good for 2 people.

Total Time

45 mins.

Ingredients

- 1 lb. beef sausage
- 8 pcs. bacon strips, chopped
- 2 cups broccoli florets
- ½ cup heavy cream
- 1 tbsp. Dijon mustard
- ¼ cup cheddar cheese, grated

Nutritional Values

- ✓ Calories: 768 kcal
- ✓ Fat: 58.96g (65%)
- ✓ Carbohydrates: 5.58g (14%)
- ✓ Protein: 46.81g (21%)
- ✓ Dietary Fiber : 8.3g
- ✓ Cholesterol: 42mg

How to Make the Dish

- ➢ Set oven at 350F.
- ➢ Cut the sausages into chunks and place on a baking dish with the chopped bacon.
- ➢ Also add the florets into the dish making sure they're equally distributed.
- ➢ In a small bowl, combine the cream and mustard and pour on top of the meat and broccoli.
- ➢ Finally, sprinkle the top of the dish with the grated cheese and bake in the oven for 35 minutes.
- ➢ Serve.

Filet Mignon Steak

Fancy a steak dinner? Here's a recipe to make an absolutely delicious steak.

Portion

This recipe to share between 4 people.

Total Time

1 hour

Ingredients

- 2 large (about 1.5 inch thick) filet mignon steaks, cut in half
- 2 tbsp. ghee
- A pinch of salt and pepper to taste

Nutritional Values

- ✓ Calories: 22 kcal
- ✓ Fat: 15.85g (64%)
- ✓ Carbohydrates: 1.06g (2%)
- ✓ Protein: 17.77g (34%)
- ✓ Dietary Fiber : 0.2g
- ✓ Cholesterol: 75mg

How to Make the Dish

- ➢ Set oven at 275F
- ➢ Take a paper towel and pat dry the steaks and then season with salt and pepper.
- ➢ Lay the steaks on a baking rack on top of a baking sheet lined with foil.
- ➢ Place in the oven to broil for 30 minutes or until the meat registers at 90F.
- ➢ Remove the steaks from the oven and then place on a skillet with ghee over high heat.
- ➢ Cook the steaks for about 2 minutes on each side.
- ➢ Reduce the heat to medium and then brown all sides for another 1 minute each.
- ➢ Serve with your favorite steak sauce.

Curried Ground Beef

If you love curry, you'll surely love this recipe. You don't have to go out to have Indian food because you can now prepare one at the comforts of your kitchen. How awesome is that?

Portion

This recipe is good for 6 people.

Total Time

30 mins.

Ingredients

- 1 lb. ground beef
- 3 pcs. carrots, chopped
- 1 pc. large tomato, chopped
- 1 tsp. mustard seeds
- 1 onion, chopped
- A handful of curry leaves
- 4 cloves of garlic, minced
- ½ tsp. ginger, minced
- 1 tsp. coriander powder
- ¼ tsp. chili powder
- ½ tsp. turmeric
- ½ tsp. sea salt
- 2 tsp. masala
- 2 tbsp. ghee
- 1 can coconut milk
- ¼ cup water

Nutritional Values

- ✓ Calories: 332 kcal
- ✓ Fat: 19.1g (52%)
- ✓ Carbohydrates: 13.9g (4%)
- ✓ Protein: 30.g (37%)
- ✓ Dietary Fiber : 3.1g
- ✓ Cholesterol: 100mg

How to Make the Dish

- ➢ Heat the ghee on a pan over medium fire.
- ➢ Throw in the mustard seeds and wait until the seeds start to pop before adding the chopped onion and curry leaves.
- ➢ Sauté for 3 minutes and then add the minced garlic and ginger. Stir and then add the rest of the spices.
- ➢ Add the ground beef and cook until brown.
- ➢ Add the chopped potato and carrots and pour the ¼ cup water. Cover and simmer for 5 minutes.
- ➢ Pour in the coconut milk, stir and cook for 15 minutes, or until the veggies are soft.
- ➢ Serve.

Aloha Burger

This is not your ordinary burger recipe as it is served with crunchy and sweet pineapples. I personally found it odd at first, but after biting into this dish, I am now a believer!

Portion

This recipe makes 4 mouthwatering patties

Total Time

30 mins.

Ingredients

- 2 lbs. ground beef
- 3 garlic cloves, minced
- 1 onion, chopped
- 1 egg yolk
- 6 whole eggs
- 6 pcs. pineapple slices
- 1 tbsp. butter
- A pinch of salt and pepper

Nutritional Values

- ✓ Calories: 451 kcal
- ✓ Fat: 55.26g (57%)
- ✓ Carbohydrates: 17.12g (7%)
- ✓ Protein: 72.39g (36%)
- ✓ Dietary Fiber : 1.2g
- ✓ Cholesterol: 1182mg

How to Make the Dish

- ➢ In a mixing bowl, combine the beef, minced garlic, chopped onion, and egg yolk. Season with salt and pepper and then combine using your hands.
- ➢ Divide the mixture into 6 equal parts and create patties.
- ➢ Grill the patties on medium heat for about 5 minutes on each side.
- ➢ Take the pineapples and then grill also for 2 minutes on each side.
- ➢ Meanwhile, melt the butter on a non-stick pan and then fry the eggs.

Serve the juicy patties with the grilled pineapple and egg on top.

Ribeye Steak in Wild Mushroom

Do you want to impress your loved ones or just have a good homemade steak? Here's a recipe I'd like to share with you that is unbelievable delicious.

Portion

This recipe is for 2 persons.

Total Time

50 mins.

Ingredients

- 2 pcs. rib eye steak (500g)
- 2 cups wild mushrooms, sliced
- 4 tbsp. plus 1 tbsp. butter
- 4 tbsp. heavy cream
- 2 tbsp. umami paste
- Salt and pepper to taste

Nutritional Values

- ✓ Calories: 945 kcal
- ✓ Fat: 81.8g (77%)
- ✓ Carbohydrates: 4g (2%)
- ✓ Protein: 49.7g (21%)
- ✓ Dietary Fiber : 0.93g

How to Make the Dish

- ➢ Generously season the steaks with salt and pepper.
- ➢ Melt the 4 tbsp. butter on a skillet over medium-high fire and cook each side for 3-4 minutes. Remember to baste the steak to get the delicious buttery taste.
- ➢ Lower the heat after 4 minutes and then cook for another 7 minutes. Set aside the steak and cover it with parchment paper to make sure it doesn't dry and remain juicy.
- ➢ Prepare the mushroom sauce by melting the 1 tbsp. butter on the same skillet heated over medium fire.
- ➢ Add the umami paste to the pan followed by the heavy cream. Whisk the ingredients for the sauce. (Add salt and pepper to your liking)
- ➢ Serve the steaks with the wild mushroom sauce.

PORK RECIPES

Sweet and Sour Baked Chops

One of my friends just love pork chops. Being a kitchen whiz, he decided to make a recipe of his own and came up with this dish.

Portion

This recipe serves 5 hungry bellies.

Total Time

1 hour 1 mins.

Ingredients

- 5 pcs. pork chops
- ½ tsp. ginger, minced
- ½ tsp. ground pepper
- ½ cup apple cider vinegar
- 2 tbsp. coconut aminos
- ½ cup erythritol
- 1 tbsp. butter

Nutritional Values

- ✓ Calories: 363 kcal
- ✓ Fat: 19.72g (49%)
- ✓ Carbohydrates: 3.49g (4%)
- ✓ Protein: 40.39g (47%)
- ✓ Dietary Fiber : 0.2g

✓ Cholesterol: 138mg

How to Make the Dish

➢ Set oven at 350F.
➢ Place all the ingredients except for the pork chop in a food processor and pulse until all the ingredients are combined.
➢ Grease a baking dish with butter and add the pork chop in it.
➢ Pour over the prepared marinade making sure that the pork chops are covered with the sauce.
➢ Place in the oven to bake for 30 minutes. Flip the pork chops over and bake for another 30 minutes.
➢ Serve.

Slow-Cooked Pulled Pork Roast

This is another recipe that will utilize your crock pot. I usually prepare this in the morning and then leave it cooking for the rest of the day so it's ready for dinner. This dish certainly tasty and will be one of your favorites (I swear!)

Portion

This recipe serves 5 persons.

Total Time

10 hours 10 mins.

Ingredients

- 1 lb. pork roast
- 3 cloves of garlic, crushed
- 1 large onion, diced
- 1 bell pepper, diced
- 2 tbsp. chili powder
- ½ tbsp. red pepper flakes
- 2 tbsp. paprika
- ½ tbsp. cumin
- 1 tsp. cayenne
- 1 tsp. kosher salt
- ¼ cup Sriracha sauce
- 1 large can roasted tomatoes

Nutritional Values

- ✓ Calories: 225 kcal
- ✓ Fat: 9.17g (36%)

✓ Carbohydrates: 10.48g (15%)
✓ Protein: 26.2g (48%)
✓ Dietary Fiber : 3.6g
✓ Cholesterol: 73mg

How to Make the Dish

➢ Place the pork at the bottom of the slow cooker.
➢ Poke 3 holes on the pork roast and insert the garlic cloves.
➢ Pour the Sriracha sauce and add the rest of the ingredients in.
➢ Cover the pot and cook for 10 hours on low.
➢ When cooked, use a fork to pull apart the pork. Serve with slices of avocado on the side.

Mom's Pork Medallions

This is a recipe I got from my mom, which I amped up by wrapping them with bacon. Doesn't this dish sound delicious?

Portion

This recipe serves 4 people.

Total Time

40 mins.

Ingredients

- 2 lb. pork medallions
- 8 strips of bacon
- 1 tsp. of each: garlic powder, dried oregano, dried basil, kosher salt
- 4 tbsp. ghee

Nutritional Values

- ✓ Calories: 656 kcal
- ✓ Fat: 40.93g (56%)
- ✓ Carbohydrates: 2.46g (1%)
- ✓ Protein: 66.39g (43%)
- ✓ Dietary Fiber : 0.4g
- ✓ Cholesterol: 181mg

How to Make the Dish

- ➢ Set oven at 400F.

- ➢ Cook the bacon on a cast iron skillet heated over medium fire. Cook for about 5-6 minutes or until the color is lightly brown. Remove the bacon from the pan and set aside.
- ➢ Combine the herbs and seasonings together in a bowl and set aside.
- ➢ Take the half cooked bacon and wrap it around the pork medallions. Secure the bacon using a toothpick.
- ➢ Rub the medallions with the seasoning mixture.
- ➢ Heat the ghee on the same skillet used to cook the bacon and cook the pork for 4-5 minutes on each side.
- ➢ Then transfer the pan into the oven and bake for 18-20 minutes. The temperature of the book should register at 145F to know when you're done.

3-Spice Pork Chop

I always have spices in my pantry and one time I thought of combining some from my stock to flavor my pork chops. Good thing it turned out tasty!

Portion

This recipe serves a group of four people.

Total Time

30 mins.

Ingredients

- 1 ½ lb. pork chops
- 1 tsp. cardamom
- 1 tsp. coriander
- 2 tsp. cumin
- ¼ cup flax seed meal
- ½ tsp. salt
- ½ tsp. pepper
- 4 tbsp. ghee

Nutritional Values

- ✓ Calories: 465 kcal
- ✓ Fat: 30.61g (59%)
- ✓ Carbohydrates: 1.35g (1%)
- ✓ Protein: 44.04g (40%)
- ✓ Dietary Fiber : 0.3g
- ✓ Cholesterol: 173mg

How to Make the Dish

- ➢ In a small bowl, combine the spices together along with the flax seed meal.
- ➢ Season the chops with salt and pepper and coat them with the spices.
- ➢ Drizzle the ghee on a skillet heated over medium fire. When hot, add the pork chops to the pan and cook for a few minutes until they turn golden brown.
- ➢ You can serve this dish with sautéed vegetables on the side.

Pork Skewers

This is a BBQ-style recipe ideal for the Ketogenic Diet. I often make this during our weekend cookouts with my friends.

Portion

This recipe makes 4-6 servings.

Total Time

20 minutes (requires at least 8 hours of marinating)

Ingredients

- 2 lb. pork shoulder, cut into cubes
- 2 cups olive oil
- 2 lemons, juiced
- 2 tbsp. balsamic vinegar
- 4 tbsp. fresh mint leaves, chopped
- 4 tbsp. fresh oregano, chopped
- 2 tsp. kosher salt
- ½ tsp. pepper

Nutritional Values

- ✓ Calories: 839kcal
- ✓ Fat: 72.5g (77%)
- ✓ Carbohydrates: 1.1g (1%)
- ✓ Protein: 43g (22)
- ✓ Dietary Fiber : 0.8g

How to Make the Dish

- ➢ Place the pork cubes on a large mixing bowl. Drizzle the olive oil over the pork and add the mint leaves, oregano, lemon juice, and balsamic vinegar. Season with salt and pepper and combine making sure that the pork is well coated with the marinade.
- ➢ Cover with a cling wrap and place in the fridge to marinate for at least 8 hours.
- ➢ Pre-heat the grill when you're ready to cook.
- ➢ Skew the pork cubes in bamboo sticks and cook on the grill for about 5-8 minutes on each side.
- ➢ Serve with green salad on the side.

Zesty Pork Sirloin

Another pork recipe with a zing! Try this dish with a salad and have a delicious and satisfying meal.

Portion

This recipe serves 4 persons.

Total Time

3 hrs. 45 mins.

Ingredients

- 1 ½ lb. pork sirloin
- ¼ tsp. garlic powder
- ¼ tsp. cumin, ground
- 3 tbsp. lime juice
- ¼ cup salsa
- 4 tbsp. butter
- A pinch of salt and pepper to taste

Nutritional Values

- ✓ Calories: 307 kcal
- ✓ Fat: 14.51g (42%)
- ✓ Carbohydrates: 3.32g (4%)
- ✓ Protein: 36.62g (55%)
- ✓ Dietary Fiber : 0.5g
- ✓ Cholesterol: 136mg

How to Make the Dish

- ➢ Combine all the spices together and then use as a rub for the pork chops.
- ➢ Melt the butter on a skillet over medium-high fire. When hot, place the pork chops in the pan and cook for 5 minutes on each side.
- ➢ In another bowl, combine the salsa and lime juice.
- ➢ Place the pork chops in a slow-cooker and top with the lime-salsa mixture.
- ➢ Cook on high for at least 3 hours.
- ➢ Serve.

Spinach Stuffed Pork Chops

Bite into this and you'll have a surprise inside—a creamy medley of feta cheese and spinach.

Portion

This recipe serves 4 persons.

Total Time

50 mins.

Ingredients

- 4 pcs. pork chops
- 1 tbsp. butter
- 2 tbsp. ghee
- 2 cups spinach
- ¼ cup feta cheese
- Salt and pepper to taste

Nutritional Values

- ✓ Calories: 386 kcal
- ✓ Fat: 22.32g (52%)
- ✓ Carbohydrates: 1.99g (2%)
- ✓ Protein: 42.22g (46%)
- ✓ Dietary Fiber : 0.5g
- ✓ Cholesterol: 148mg

How to Make the Dish

> ➢ Melt the butter in a skillet over medium fire. Add the spinach, season with salt and pepper. When almost done, add the feta cheese and continue to cook until wilted. Set aside.
> ➢ Preheat oven at 350F.
> ➢ Using a sharp knife, cut a slit on the pork chop to create a pocket for the filling. Stuff the pork chops with the spinach and feta mixture.
> ➢ Heat the 2 tbsp. ghee on a skillet over medium heat and fry the pork for about 4-5 minutes on each side.
> ➢ Transfer the pan into the oven and bake for another 20 minutes.
> ➢ Serve.

SEAFOOD RECIPES

Easy Salmon Salad with Avocado

This is a recipe I always make for a light lunch or dinner—or when I'm too lazy to cook!

Portion

This recipe makes 2 salad servings.

Total Time

40 mins.

Ingredients

- 1 pc. salmon fillet
- 1 pc. green onion, chopped
- 2 tbsp. lime juice
- ¼ cup keto mayo
- 2 tbsp. fresh dill
- 1 tbsp. ghee
- 1 avocado
- Pinch of salt and pepper

Nutritional Values

- ✓ Calories: 490 kcal
- ✓ Fat: 31.99g (57%)
- ✓ Carbohydrates: 30.21g (14%)
- ✓ Protein: 26.7g (26%)
- ✓ Dietary Fiber : 9.3g
- ✓ Cholesterol: 94mg

How to Make the Dish

- ➢ Set oven at 400F.
- ➢ Lay the salmon fillet on a baking sheet lined with parchment paper. Drizzle with juice of lime and ghee on top.
- ➢ Season the salmon with salt and pepper and place in the oven to bake for 25 minutes.
- ➢ When cooked, pull the salmon meat using a fork and place in a bowl.
- ➢ Add the mayo and green onions in the bowl and stir.
- ➢ Mash the avocado and add to the salmon salad. Lightly toss the ingredients together and serve.

Salmon Fillets

Here's another salmon recipe I'd like to share with you. This baked salmon is full of herbs and spices making it full of flavor. Who says healthy food isn't delicious?

Portion

This recipe serves 3 persons.

Total Time

25 mins. (plus 4 hours for marinating)

Ingredients

- 1 lb. salmon fillet
- ¼ cup button mushrooms, chopped
- 1 clove of garlic, minced
- ½ cup scallions, chopped
- ¼ cup tamari
- ¼ tsp. rosemary
- ¼ tsp. thyme
- ¼ tsp. tarragon
- ¼ tsp. basil
- ¼ tsp. oregano
- ¼ tsp. ginger, ground
- 2 tbsp. butter

Nutritional Values

- ✓ Calories: 323 kcal
- ✓ Fat: 18.62g (51%)
- ✓ Carbohydrates: 3.35g (4%)

✓ Protein: 34.46g (45%)
✓ Dietary Fiber : 0.8g
✓ Cholesterol: 122mg

How to Make the Dish

➤ Set oven at 350F.
➤ Place the fish fillet in a re-sealable plastic bag and pour over the tamari, coconut oil, as well as the herbs and spices. Shake the bag well to coat the fish with the sauce and marinate in the fridge for 4 hours.
➤ When done marinating, place the salmon fillet on a baking sheet lined with foil and bake for at least 10 minutes.
➤ Melt the butter on a pan over medium heat. Add the mushrooms and scallions into the pan and cook until tender.
➤ Take the salmon out from the oven and pour over the sautéed mushrooms. Place the fish back in the oven to bake for another 10 mins. Serve.

Parmesan Crusted Fish

This dish is one of my favorite things to order whenever I go to a restaurant nearby my house. One day I stumbled over this recipe and made a version of my own.

Portion

This recipe serves 4 persons.

Total Time

40 mins.

Ingredients

- 1 lb. cream dory fillet
- 2 tbsp. milk
- 1 egg
- ¼ cup parmesan cheese, grated
- 2 tbsp. almond flour
- ½ tsp. smoked paprika
- Pinch of salt and pepper to taste

Nutritional Values

- ✓ Calories: 293 kcal
- ✓ Fat: 26.65g (80%)
- ✓ Carbohydrates: 6.99g (9%)
- ✓ Protein: 7.71g (11%)
- ✓ Dietary Fiber : 0.3g
- ✓ Cholesterol: 236mg

How to Make the Dish

- ➤ Set the oven at 350F
- ➤ Whisk the egg and milk together in a bowl.
- ➤ In a re-sealable plastic bag combine all the dry ingredients and shake well.
- ➤ Dip the fish fillet into the egg and milk mixture and place inside the plastic bag. Shake to cover the fillets with the breading.
- ➤ Place the fish fillets on a baking sheet lined with foil and cook in the oven for 25 minutes.
- ➤ Serve with lemon wedges on the side.

Fish in Orange Pecan Butter Sauce

I like eating fish and so I have plenty of fish recipes up my sleeve. This one is a recipe I discovered when I was looking for ways to cook trout.

Portion

This recipe makes 4 servings.

Total Time

25 mins.

Ingredients

- 1 pc. trout fillet, skin on
- ½ cup pecan nuts, chopped
- 1 pc. orange, juiced and zested
- 2 tbsp. butter, divided
- 1 tbsp. parsley, chopped
- A pinch of salt and pepper to taste

Nutritional Values

- ✓ Calories: 350 kcal
- ✓ Fat: 33.01g (81%)
- ✓ Carbohydrates: 5.66g 65%)
- ✓ Protein: 10.87g (13%)
- ✓ Dietary Fiber : 2.8g
- ✓ Cholesterol: 38mg

How to Make the Dish

- ➢ Melt 1 tbsp. of butter on a cast iron skillet over medium fire.
- ➢ Flavor the trout with salt and pepper and place on the hot pan with the skin side up.
- ➢ Sear the fish for 3 minutes on the other side. Set aside.
- ➢ Using the same pan, melt the remaining butter and add the chopped pecans for about a minute. Pour the orange juice and allow to simmer for 2 minutes.
- ➢ Orange pecan sauce over the fish and sprinkle with the orange zest and chopped parsley. Serve.

Grilled Fish

Basic—this is what this meal is. But don't let its simplicity fool you as you will definitely love this one!

Portion

This recipe serves 4 persons.

Total Time

30 mins.

Ingredients

- 1 lb. tilapia fillets
- 2 limes, juiced
- 1 tbsp. fresh parsley, chopped
- 1 tsp. dill
- ¼ tsp. smoked paprika
- A pinch of salt and pepper to taste
- 2 tbsp. butter

Nutritional Values

- ✓ Calories: 171 kcal
- ✓ Fat: 7.7g (40%)
- ✓ Carbohydrates: 3.06g (5%)
- ✓ Protein: 23.2g (54%)
- ✓ Dietary Fiber : 0.3g
- ✓ Cholesterol: 72mg

How to Make the Dish

- ➤ Place a fillet on top of one heavy duty foil.
- ➤ Melt the butter in a saucepan heated over low fire. Pour the lemon juice, add the dill, parsley, salt and pepper.
- ➤ Equally pour the butter on top of the fillets and season with paprika on top.
- ➤ Wrap the fillets with the foil making sure it's secured. Cook on the grill for 5 minutes on each side.
- ➤ Serve.

Buttered Shrimp

Shrimp in garlicky, butter sauce, what else can you ask for?

Portion

This recipe serves 4 persons.

Total Time

15 mins.

Ingredients

- 1 ½ lb. shrimp, peel and veins removed
- 2 tbsp. plus 6 tbsp. butter
- 4 cloves of garlic, minced
- 1 juice of lemon
- ¼ cup low-sodium chicken stock
- A pinch of salt and pepper
- 2 tbsp. fresh parsley, chopped

Nutritional Values

- ✓ Calories: 236 kcal
- ✓ Fat: 25.52 (58%)
- ✓ Carbohydrates: 3.2g (3%)
- ✓ Protein: 35.79g (39%)
- ✓ Dietary Fiber : 0.3g
- ✓ Cholesterol: 490mg

How to Make the Dish

- ➢ Place a skillet over medium fire and melt the butter.

> ➢ Add the shrimps and season with salt and pepper. Stir and cook for about 3 minutes or until the shrimps turn pink. Set aside.
> ➢ Using the same pan, sauté the garlic for 1 minute. Pour the chicken stock and juice of lemon and allow to simmer for 3-5 minutes.
> ➢ Add the 6 tbsp. butter on to the pan and stir until it fully melts.
> ➢ Add the shrimp back to the pan and toss to coat with the garlic butter sauce.
> ➢ Garnish with chopped parsley on top before serving.

Creamy Shrimp and Bacon Bowl

Shrimps are delicious as they are, but this recipe is much more mouthwatering as it is served with crispy bacon and creamy sauce.

Portion

This recipe is good for a group of 4.

Total Time

35 mins.

Ingredients

- ¼ lb. shrimps, peel and vein removed
- ¼ lb. smoked salmon, roughly chopped
- 4 bacon strips, roughly chopped
- 1 cup button mushrooms, sliced
- ½ cup coconut cream
- A pinch of salt and pepper

Nutritional Values

- ✓ Calories: 340 kcal
- ✓ Fat: 29g (86.5%)
- ✓ Carbohydrates: 3.5g (9%)
- ✓ Protein: 17g (4.5%)
- ✓ Dietary Fiber : 1g

How to Make the Dish

- ➢ Cook the chopped bacon on a cast iron skillet over medium fire.
- ➢ Add the sliced mushrooms when the bacon is almost crispy and then cook for another 5 minutes. Remember to stir constantly.
- ➢ Add the salmon to the pan and cook for 2 minutes.
- ➢ Then, add the deveined shrimp and allow to cook for another 2 minutes.
- ➢ Pour the coconut cream on the pan and then set the heat to low fire. Allow to simmer for a minute.
- ➢ Serve.

Baked Sardines

This recipe couldn't be much easier. Newbies in the kitchen can totally ace this.

Portion

This recipe serves 4 persons.

Total Time

25 minutes

Ingredients

- 800g sardines
- 1 tsp. kosher salt
- A pinch of black pepper
- 8 tbsp. extra virgin olive oil
- 4 tbsp. mint leaves, chopped
- 4 tsp. dried basil

Nutritional Values

- ✓ Calories: 482 kcal
- ✓ Fat: 40g (69.1%)
- ✓ Carbohydrates: 0.20g (0.2%)
- ✓ Protein: 40.01g (30.8%)
- ✓ Dietary Fiber : 0.22g

How to Make the Dish

- ➢ Set the oven at 350F.
- ➢ Season sardines with salt and pepper and place on a baking rack.
- ➢ Bake in the oven for 10 minutes.
- ➢ When done cooking, sprinkle the sardines with the mint leaves and basil and finally, drizzle with extra virgin olive oil.

Tuna Salad

Besides salmon, tuna is another personal favorite when it comes to eating it with salad. Here's another quick fish and salad recipe.

Portion

This recipe makes a large bowl of tuna salad.

Total Time

5 minutes

Ingredients

- 1 head of romaine lettuce
- 1 can tuna
- 2 hardboiled eggs, sliced
- 2 tbsp. chives, chopped
- 2 tbsp. mayonnaise
- 1 tbsp. lime juice
- 1 tbsp. olive oil
- Pinch of salt to taste

Nutritional Values

- ✓ Calories: 996 kcal
- ✓ Fat: 45.83g (56%)
- ✓ Carbohydrates: 25.08g (12%)
- ✓ Protein: 59.75g (32%)
- ✓ Dietary Fiber : 13.7g
- ✓ Cholesterol: 1297mg

How to Make the Dish

➢ Tear the lettuce and place on a serving plate.
➢ In a bowl, combine the tuna, mayo, lime juice, and olive oil. Season with salt and toss to coat the fish well with the dressing.
➢ Serve the tuna on top of the bed of lettuce and top with the slices of egg on top.

Salmon and Avocado Omelet

Don't think that omelets are just for breakfast only. Here is a recipe with salmon and avocado. Delicious!

Portion

This recipe serves 2 persons.

Total Time

30 mins.

Ingredients

- 3 whole eggs
- 50g smoked salmon
- ½ avocado, sliced
- 2 tbsp. cream cheese
- 2 tbsp. chives, chopped
- 1 tbsp. butter
- A pinch of salt and pepper to taste

Nutritional Values

- ✓ Calories: 765 kcal
- ✓ Fat: 66.9g (78%)
- ✓ Carbohydrates: 13.3g (3%)
- ✓ Protein: 36.9g (19%)
- ✓ Dietary Fiber : 7.4g

How to Make the Dish

- ➤ Whisk the eggs in a bowl and season with salt and pepper.
- ➤ In a separate bowl, combine the cream cheese and chives together. Set aside.
- ➤ Melt the butter in a non-stick pan over medium heat. Pour the egg and move the pan side to side. Cook until done.
- ➤ Transfer the cooked egg into a plate and spread the cream cheese and chive mixture on top.
- ➤ Add the smoked salmon on top along with the avocado slices. Fold to create an omelet.
- ➤ Serve.

Slow Cooked Lobster Bisque

Don't be intimate by this dish, it's even quite easy to prepare!

Portion

This recipe serves 4 persons.

Total Time

4 hours

Ingredients

- 4 pcs. lobster tails
- 1 clove of garlic
- 2 pcs. shallots, minced
- ¼ cup fresh parsley leaves, chopped
- 1 tsp. dill
- ½ tsp. smoked paprika
- ¼ tsp. ground pepper
- 2 cups heavy cream
- 4 cups low-sodium chicken broth
- 1 can diced tomatoes (with juice)

Nutritional Values

- ✓ Calories: 505 kcal
- ✓ Fat: 24.96g (58%)
- ✓ Carbohydrates: 7.12g (7%)
- ✓ Protein: 31.44g (35%)
- ✓ Dietary Fiber: 1.2g
- ✓ Cholesterol: 273mg

How to Make the Dish

- ➢ Place the minced garlic and shallot in a bowl and microwave on high for 2 minutes.
- ➢ Transfer into a slow cooker and then add the rest of the ingredients except for the lobster tails and heavy cream.
- • Cut the end of the lobster tail and then add to the crockpot. Cook on high for 3 hours.

- ➢ When done cooking, remove the lobster tails from the pot and use an immersion blender to puree the soup. This depends on the consistency you prefer your bisque to be.
- ➢ Add the lobster back into the pot and cook for another 45 minutes.
- ➢ Remove again the lobster and chop.
- ➢ Pour the heavy cream into the pot along with the chopped lobster. Stir well and serve hot.

Mussels in Parsley Butter Sauce

I like my seafood cooked simple. Here is an easy recipe of mussels in delicious butter sauce.

Portion

This recipe makes 4 servings.

Total Time

35 minutes

Ingredients

- 2 lbs. mussels
- 4 cloves of garlic, chopped
- 2 pcs. shallots, chopped
- 2 cups white wine
- 4 tbsp. parsley, chopped
- 4 pcs. bay leaves
- 8 tbsp. ghee
- 1 tbsp. butter

Nutritional Values

- ✓ Calories: 207 kcal
- ✓ Fat: 12.9g (65.5%)
- ✓ Carbohydrates: 4.6g (10.3%)
- ✓ Protein: 10.7g (24.2%)
- ✓ Dietary Fiber : 0.25g

How to Make the Dish

- ➤ Wash the mussels over cold water, making sure they're clean.
- ➤ Melt the butter on a pot over medium fire and sauté the garlic, onion, and bay leaves.
- ➤ Pour the white wine in the pot and bring to a boil.
- ➤ Add the mussels to the pot, stir and cover. Cook for 5 minutes.
- ➤ Meanwhile, place the ghee in a bowl and heat in the microwave. Add parsley, stir and Set aside.
- ➤ Place the cooked mussels on a serving dish and pour over the butter and parsley sauce. Serve.

SNACK RECIPES

Double Chocolate Chip Cookies

Great snack anytime for a quick energy boost!

Portion

This recipe serves 4 persons (30 cookies).

Total Time

30 minutes

Ingredients

- 4 tbsp. Cocoa Powder
- 3 eggs
- 1¼ tsp vanilla extract
- 400g macadamia butter
- 90g natvia
- 1 cup Sugar free chocolate chips
- 1 tsp Baking Powder
- 1 cup golden flax meal

Nutritional Values

- ✓ Calories: 156kcal
- ✓ Fat: 14g (88.7%)
- ✓ Carbohydrates: 6g (2.8%)
- ✓ Protein: 3g (8.5%)
- ✓ Dietary Fiber : 5g
- ✓ Cholesterol: mg

How to Make the Snack

> ➤ Pre Heat the ingredients at 375F in Oven
> ➤ Retrieve and mix the ingredients thoroughly with a food mixer.
> ➤ Create 30 tablespoon sized balls and press onto a lined baking tray.
> ➤ Bake cookies for 15 – 20 minutes.
> ➤ Cookies will be ready to serve once solidify.

Avocado Chocolate Pudding

One of my favourites! Delicious and healthy combo.

Portion

This recipe serves 2 persons.

Total Time

10 minutes

Ingredients

- 1 tbsp. coconut milk
- 1 avocado
- 2½ tbsp. raw cocoa powder
- 1 pinch sea salt
- ½ tbsp. vanilla extract
- 1 tsp ceylon cinnamon
- 1 tbsp coconut sugar
- 1 pinch stevia
- 1/16 tsp ground cayenne pepper

Nutritional Values

- ✓ Calories: 180 kcal
- ✓ Fat: 15g (84.9%)
- ✓ Carbohydrates: 3.5g (7.6%)
- ✓ Protein: 3g (7.5%)

How to Make the Snack

- ➤ Cut and pit the avocado into a blender.
- ➤ Blend until smooth.
- ➤ Add in the coconut milk, cocoa powder and vanilla extract. Blend until smooth.
- ➤ Add in coconut sugar, cayenne pepper, stevia and cinnamon.
- ➤ Continue blending and make sure that all the chunks are blended by scraping down the sides of the food processor.
- ➤ Serve with sprinkle of sea salt on the pudding.

Crunchy Kale Chips

Easy to prepare for quick healthy bites.

Portion

This recipe serves 2 persons.

Total Time

20 minutes

Ingredients

- 1 tsp soy sauce
- 1 tsp fish sauce
- 2 tbsp sriracha
- 2 tbsp olive oil
- 1 bunch of kale
- 1tsp of sea salt

Nutritional Values

- ✓ Calories: 49 kcal
- ✓ Fat: 0.9g (12%)
- ✓ Carbohydrates: 9g (72%)
- ✓ Protein: 4.3g (16%)
- ✓ Dietary Fiber : 1g
- ✓ Cholesterol: 0mg

How to Make the Snack

- ➢ Remove the kale from the stems
- ➢ Preheat oven to 350 F
- ➢ Line with parchment paper
- ➢ Break it into chip sized pieces and placed it in a bowl.

- ➢ Add sriracha, olive oil, soy sauce and fish sauce.
- ➢ Swirl the mixture and pour the dressing over the kale leaves.
- ➢ Place the leaves out on the parchment paper
- ➢ Baked until crisp. Approx. 8 – 12 minutes.
- ➢ Sprinkling the sea salt over the kale leaves
- ➢ Serve it.

Granola Bars

Handy keto bars for on the go need!

Portion

This recipe serves 10 bars.

Total Time

30 minutes

Ingredients

- 2 eggs
- 1 tbsp. nut butter
- 2 tsp dried cinnamon
- 2 tbsp. cocoa nibs
- 1 tsp vanilla
- 50g shredded coconut
- 100g almonds
- 50g pumpkin seeds
- 50g linseed
- 50g sunflower seeds
- 50g pumpkin seeds
- 50g macadamia nuts
- 3 tbsp. stevia
- 50g coconut oil

Nutritional Values

- ✓ Calories: 245 kcal
- ✓ Fat: 21g (77%)
- ✓ Carbohydrates: 7g (11%)
- ✓ Protein: 7g (11%)

✓ Dietary Fiber : 4.5g
✓ Cholesterol: 0mg

How to Make the Snack

➢ Mix all the ingredients into the blender
➢ Blend until smooth but little chunks of nuts and seeds are still visible.
➢ Form 10 bars and place it on a dish with lined parchment paper
➢ Bake at 350F until golden or for 20 minutes.

Pepper Sea Salt Pork Rinds

Another fat bomb that you should have in your kitchen.

Portion

This recipe serves 2 persons.

Total Time

30 minutes

Ingredients

- Pinch sea salt
- Pepper
- 2 to 4 lbs pork back fat and skin
- coconut oil

Nutritional Values

- ✓ Calories: 152 kcal
- ✓ Fat: 20g (100%)
- ✓ Carbohydrates: 0g (0%)
- ✓ Protein: 0g (0%)
- ✓ Dietary Fiber : 1g
- ✓ Cholesterol: 0mg

How to Make the Snack

- ➢ Preheat oven to 250F
- ➢ Slice the pork skin and fat into long strips carefully. A sharp knife is required.
- ➢ Separate a portion of the fat from the skin from one end of the strip.
- ➢ Slice further to remove remaining fat.

- ➢ Cut each strip into squares.
- ➢ Place the strip (fat-side) down, on the wire rack with a baking sheet beneath.
- ➢ Bake until the skin is crisp. Approx. 3 hours.
- ➢ Pour the coconut oil into the pan.
- ➢ Heat up the oil.
- ➢ Add the pork rinds and cook until they puff up. Approx. 3 – 5 minutes.
- ➢ Drain on a paper towel-lined plate.
- ➢ Serve with sprinkle of pepper and sea salt.

Salted Crispy Macadamia Nuts

Unbelievable easy to prepare! Tasty!

Portion

This recipe serves 4 persons.

Total Time

15 minutes

Ingredients

- 3lb raw macadamia nuts
- 3 tbsp. sea salt
- filtered water

Nutritional Values

- ✓ Calories: 945kcal
- ✓ Fat: 100g (89%)
- ✓ Carbohydrates: 17g (7%)
- ✓ Protein: 10g (4%)
- ✓ Dietary Fiber : 11g
- ✓ Cholesterol: 0mg

How to Make the Snack

- ➢ Mix the nuts and sea salt in a bowl and cover by 3 inches of water
- ➢ Leave the bowl in a warm area for 8 hours.
- ➢ Drain the nuts, and put them back in the bowl.
- ➢ Add another few teaspoons of sea salt to season.
- ➢ Place the nuts in your oven on lowest setting until dried out.

Hard Boiled Egg

Simply egg! It's that simple! Keto Quickie!

Portion

This recipe serves 2 persons.

Total Time

10 minutes

Ingredients

- 4 eggs

Nutritional Values

- ✓ Calories: 202 kcal
- ✓ Fat: 14g (62%)
- ✓ Carbohydrates: 2g (3%)
- ✓ Protein: 17g (35%)
- ✓ Dietary Fiber : 0g
- ✓ Cholesterol: 373mg

How to Make the Snack

- ➢ Place the eggs into a pot.
- ➢ Cover it with water with the eggs submerge.
- ➢ Boil over medium-high heat
- ➢ Place lid over the pot
- ➢ Remove and let it cool for 10 minutes.
- ➢ Serve it.

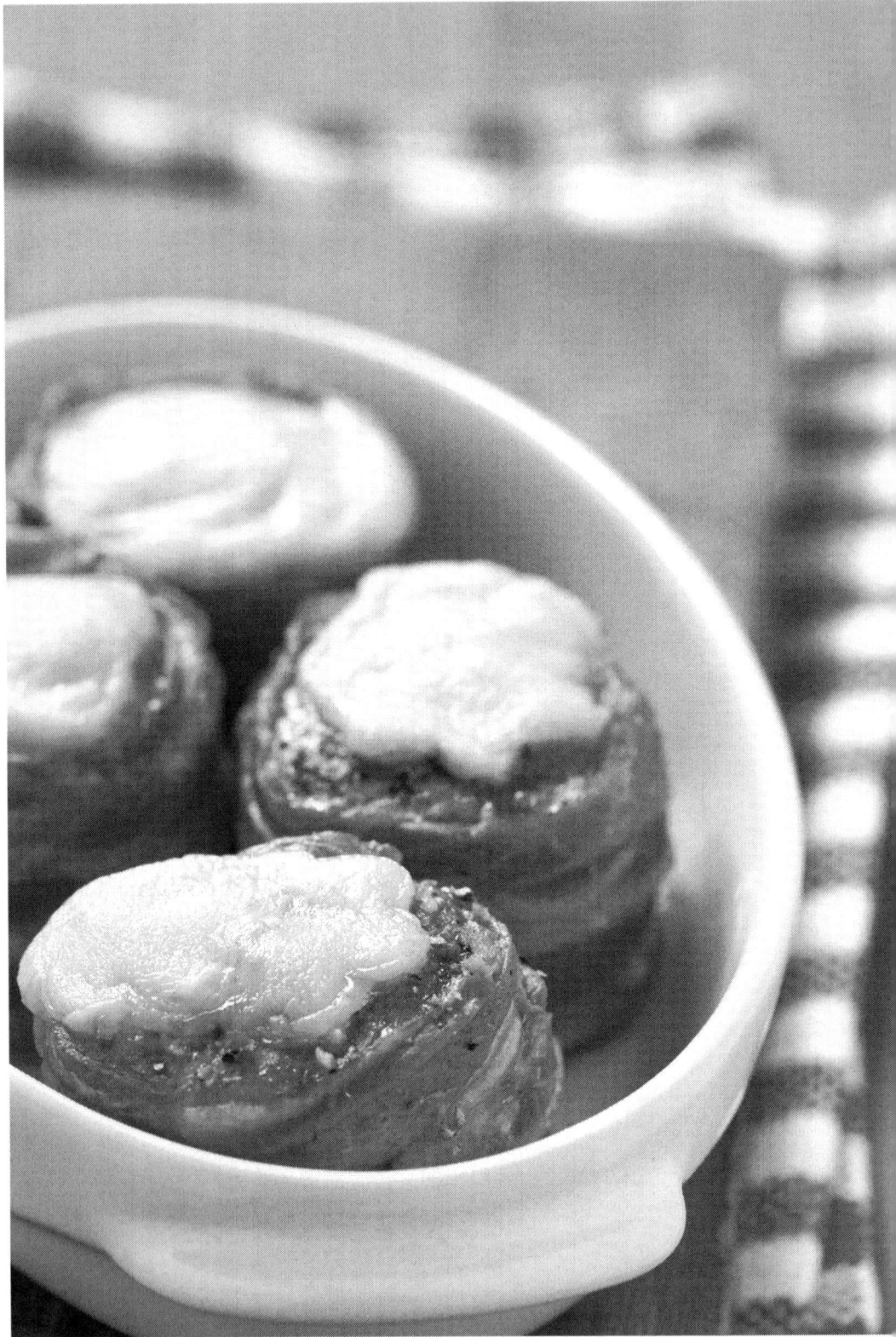

Cheesy Bacon Wrap Sticks

Delicious Cheese with Bacon! You can't go wrong with that!

Portion

This recipe serves 2 persons.

Total Time

15 minutes

Ingredients

- 4 slices of bacon
- coconut oil
- 2 mozzarella cheese sticks
- 1 egg

Nutritional Values

- ✓ Calories: 113 kcal
- ✓ Fat: 9g (72%)
- ✓ Carbohydrates: 1g (3%)
- ✓ Protein: 7g (25%)
- ✓ Dietary Fiber : 0g
- ✓ Cholesterol: mg

How to Make the Snack

- ➤ Beat the egg in a bowl
- ➤ Slice the cheese stick into quarters.
- ➤ Preheat coconut oil in deep fryer to 350 F
- ➤ Dip the ends of the bacon into the bowl.
- ➤ Wrap the cheese sticks with bacon.

➤ Drop the bacon wrapped cheese into the deep fryer
➤ Cook until the bacon is brown and crispy. Approx. 2 – 3 minutes.
➤ Transfer over to a plate with paper towel.
➤ Serve it.

Fried Avocado with Lemon

Must try!

Portion

This recipe serves 2 persons.

Total Time

7 minutes

Ingredients

- 1 avocado
- 1 tbsp. lemon juice
- 1 tbsp. coconut oil
- pinch of sea salt

Nutritional Values

- ✓ Calories: 180 kcal
- ✓ Fat: 18g (89%)
- ✓ Carbohydrates: 9g (7%)
- ✓ Protein: 3g (4%)
- ✓ Dietary Fiber : 7g
- ✓ Cholesterol: 0mg

How to Make the Snack

- ➢ Remove the seed and slice the avocado into pieces
- ➢ Preheat the pan with coconut oil
- ➢ Fry the avocado slices till gentle brown.
- ➢ Sprinkle the lemon juice and sea salt over the slices.
- ➢ Serve it.

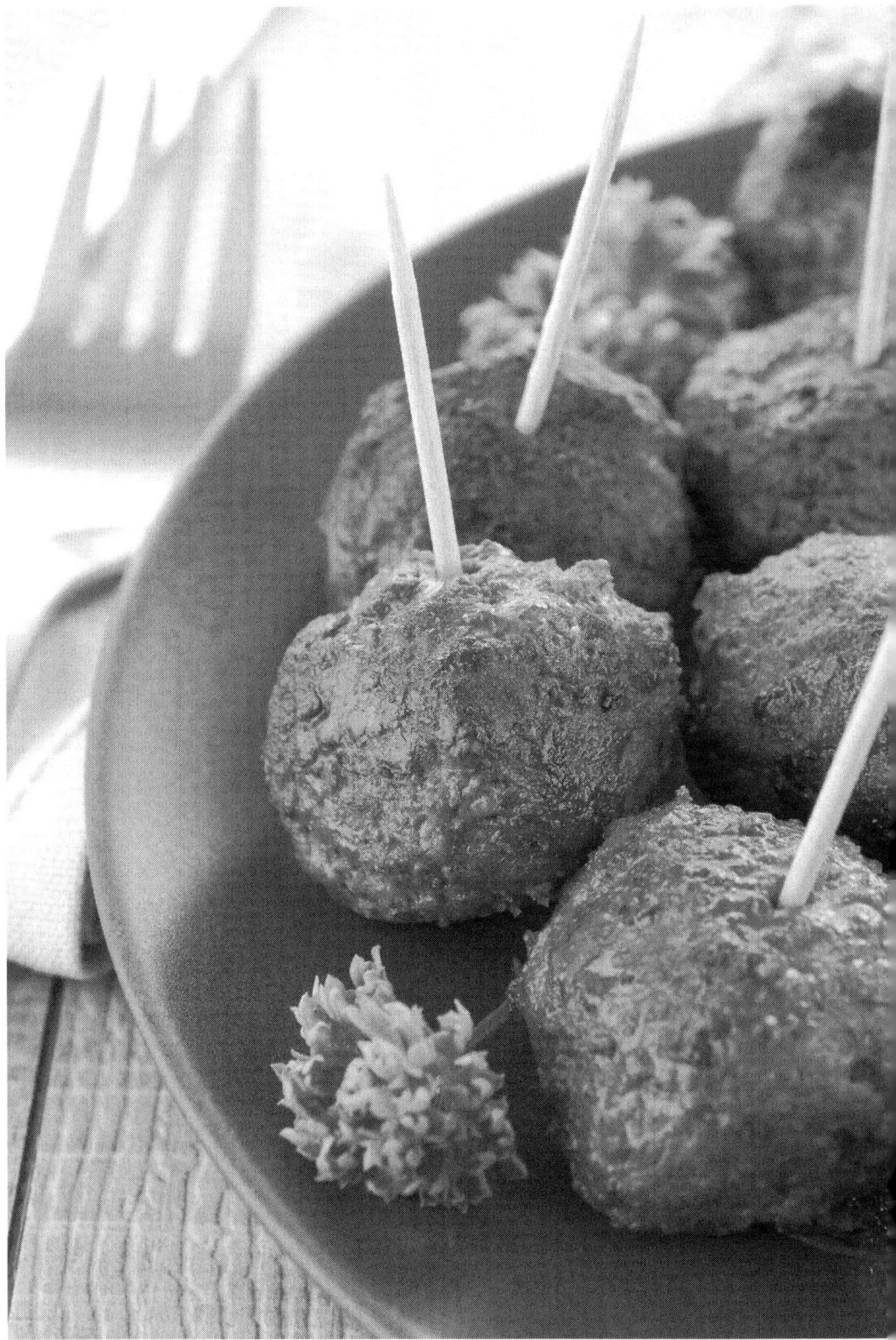

Keto Meatballs

The meatballs are great for a keto party!

Portion

This recipe serves 4 persons. (20 – 25 meatballs)

Total Time

30 minutes

Ingredients

- 500g ground beef
- 2 eggs
- 1 tsp dried tyme
- 1 tsp sea salt
- 2 cloves garlic, minced
- 1 tsp dried oregano
- coconut flour
- 1 cup diced mozzarella
- freshly grounded black pepper
- ½ cup coconut flour

Nutritional Values

- ✓ Calories: 117kcal
- ✓ Fat: 9.3g (73%)
- ✓ Carbohydrates: 1.4g (3%)
- ✓ Protein: 7g (24%)
- ✓ Dietary Fiber : 0.5g
- ✓ Cholesterol: mg

How to Make the Snack

- ➢ Preheat the over to 450F
- ➢ Dice the mozzarella in 20 -25 square pieces
- ➢ Place it in freezer for 45 - 60 minutes
- ➢ Combine all the ingredients into a large bowl.
- ➢ Mix and Stir with your clean hands
- ➢ Roll the meat into 20 – 25 pieces
- ➢ Remove the cheese from freezer
- ➢ Wrap the meat over the cheese.
- ➢ Roll between hands and placed it on the baking tray with parchment paper.
- ➢ Bake for 13 – 15 minutes.
- ➢ Serve it.

DESSERT RECIPES

Keto Almond Coffee Ice Cream

How about a coffee ice cream to go along as your dessert?

Portion

This recipe serves 4 persons.

Total Time

30 minutes

Ingredients

- ½ cup almond milk
- 4 egg yolks
- ⅛ tsp sea salt
- ¼ cup coffee beans
- ¼ cup granulated sugar
- ½ tsp vanilla extract
- 2 cups organic whipping cream
- almond nuts

Nutritional Values

- ✓ Calories: 359 kcal
- ✓ Fat: 35g (86%)
- ✓ Carbohydrates: 1g (1%)
- ✓ Protein: 2g (2%)
- ✓ Dietary Fiber : 2g
- ✓ Cholesterol: mg

How to Make the Dessert

- ➤ Crunch the almond nuts into smaller pieces with blender
- ➤ Mix whipping cream, coffee beans and almond milk into a bowl.
- ➤ Seal and soak it overnight.
- ➤ Heat the mixture in the microwave for 2 minutes.
- ➤ Remove the beans
- ➤ Add sea salt, vanilla, granulated sugar and egg yolks.
- ➤ Stir well.
- ➤ Microwave for another 30 seconds and Stir. Do it 3 times.
- ➤ Once mixture has thicken, pour it through a sieve to remove any lumps.
- ➤ Chill overnight in freezer.
- ➤ Run the custard through an ice cream maker.
- ➤ Sprinkle the crunched almond nuts.
- ➤ Serve it.

Keto Peanut Butter Popsicles

Popsicles is fun! Easy to prepare!

Portion

This recipe serves group of 6 people.

Total Time

10 minutes

Ingredients

- 1 cup peanut butter
- ½ vanilla extract
- 1 cup whipping cream
- ¼ cup granulated sugar
- ¼ cup swerve
- 8 oz. cream cheese
- 4 oz. baking unsweetened chocolate
- 4 pkts Stevia

Nutritional Values

- ✓ Calories: 203kcal
- ✓ Fat: 18g (82%)
- ✓ Carbohydrates: 11g (8%)
- ✓ Protein: 5g (10%)
- ✓ Dietary Fiber : 7g
- ✓ Cholesterol: 24mg

How to Make the Dessert

- ➢ Mix the peanut butter, vanilla extract, whipping cream, granulated sugar, swerve, cream cheese together.

- ➢ Spoon the mixture into popsicle molds
- ➢ Place a popsicle stick into each mold.
- ➢ Freeze 6 hours or overnight
- ➢ Remove the popsicles by running the mold under hot water.
- ➢ Melt the baking chocolate and add Stevia.
- ➢ Dip the popsicle in the chocolate.
- ➢ Place the dipped popsicles on a parchment paper to cool.
- ➢ Place the dipped popsicles in freezer.
- ➢ Serve it.

Yummy Brownies

Savoury brownies for the needed boost.

Portion

This recipe serves group of 12.

Total Time

35 minutes

Ingredients

Brownies
- ¾ cup granulated erythritol
- ½ cup coconut flour
- ½ cup butter ghee
- 2 tbsp cocoa powder
- 3 eggs
- 1tsp baking soda
- ½ cup brewed organic coffee
- 6 tbsp. unsweetened almond milk
- 1¼ tsp apple cider vinegar
- 1 tsp vanilla extract

Frosting
- ¼ coconut oil
- 1½ tbsp unsweetened almond milk
- ½ tsp organic vanilla extract
- ½ cup erythritol
- 1 tbsp cocoa powder

Nutritional Values

- ✓ Calories: 171kcal
- ✓ Fat: 16g (92%)
- ✓ Carbohydrates: 2g (1%)
- ✓ Protein: 3g (7%)
- ✓ Dietary Fiber : 2.2g
- ✓ Cholesterol: mg

How to Make the Dessert

- ➢ Preheat oven at 400F
- ➢ Oil the pan well
- ➢ Mix the coconut flour and erythritol together in a bowl. Set aside.
- ➢ Mix butter ghee with brewed coffee and cocoa powder. Stir and heat to boiling on stove top.
- ➢ Combine both mix and Stir well.
- ➢ Add 3 eggs, almond milk, baking soda, vanilla extract and apple cider vinegar mixture into the combined mixture.
- ➢ Use an electric mixer to mix them together.
- ➢ Pour the mixture into the pan.
- ➢ Bake at 400F for 20 minutes
- ➢ Prepare the frosting by mixing the butter ghee, almond milk and cocoa powder in a saucepan.
- ➢ Stir and heat to a boil. Change to lowest heat.
- ➢ Add erythritol and vanilla extract. Stir well. Maintain lowest heat.
- ➢ Pour warm frosting over the brownies. Use spoon to spread.
- ➢ Cool brownies and frosting.
- ➢ Place it in the fridge for further cooling. Approx. 1 hour.
- ➢ Slice and Serve it.

Keto Lemon Curd

Lemon curd is one of my favorites!

Portion

This recipe serves 1 person.

Total Time

15 minutes

Ingredients

- 2 organic eggs
- 2 organic egg yolks
- 3tbsp. granulated erythritol
- 6 tbsp. butter cubes
- ½ cup organic lemon juice

Nutritional Values

- ✓ Calories: 200kcal
- ✓ Fat: 20g (90%)
- ✓ Carbohydrates: 1g (4%)
- ✓ Protein: 3g (6%)
- ✓ Dietary Fiber : 0g
- ✓ Cholesterol: 60mg

How to Make the Dessert

- ➢ Mix the lemon juice, erythritol, egg and egg yolks together in a pan.
- ➢ Add the butter cubes and turn on the stove and adjust to lowest heat

➢ Stir well
➢ Once the butter melts, turn the heat up to medium-high
➢ Stir until thicken.
➢ Pour the mix over a sieve or mesh strainer to remove any egg bits.
➢ Place it in fridge.

Low Carb Cheesecake Brownie

Savour dessert combo that makes the day better!

Portion

This recipe serves 5 persons.

Total Time

30 minutes

Ingredients

Cheesecake Filling
- 2 eggs
- ¼ cup heavy cream
- ½ cup granulated erythritol
- ½ tsp vanilla extract
- 1 lb cream cheese, softened

Brownie
- 2 eggs
- ¼ cup cocoa powder
- pinch sea salt
- ¼ cup chopped walnuts
- ¼ tsp vanilla
- ¾ cup granulated erythritol
- ½ cup butter
- 2 oz. unsweetened chocolate
- ½ cup almond flour

Nutritional Values

- ✓ Calories: 381 kcal
- ✓ Fat: 34g (84%)
- ✓ Carbohydrates: 7g (6%)
- ✓ Protein: 9g (10%)
- ✓ Dietary Fiber : 2g
- ✓ Cholesterol: 156mg

How to Make the Dessert

- ➢ Preheat oven to 325F
- ➢ Butter the sauce pan and wrap the bottom with foil
- ➢ Melt butter and chocolate in the microwave oven in 30 seconds interval until smooth.
- ➢ Mix the sea salt, almond flour and cocoa powder in a small bowl.
- ➢ Beat eggs with erythritol and vanilla until smooth in a bowl.
- ➢ Add the almond flour and beat it
- ➢ Add the butter chocolate mixture and beat it till smooth.
- ➢ Stir well
- ➢ Spread evenly over bottom of prepared pan.
- ➢ Bake 15 to 20 minutes until it is soft in the center.
- ➢ Set aside to cool for 20 minutes
- ➢ For Cheesecake filling, reduce to 300F
- ➢ Beat cream cheese until smooth.
- ➢ Beat eggs with erythritol and vanilla until smooth in a bowl.
- ➢ Pour filling over crust and place the cheesecake on a bake sheet.
- ➢ Bake until edges are set and center is soft. Approx. 35 – 45 minutes.
- ➢ Remove from oven and cool down.
- ➢ Loosen the edge with knife.
- ➢ Cover with plastic wrap and refrigerate for 3 hours.
- ➢ Serve it.

Coconut Oil Candies

Quick easy bite to get the occasional keto boost.

Portion

This recipe serves 2 persons.

Total Time

15 minutes

Ingredients

- 4 tbsp unsweetened cocoa powder
- 1 cup softened cold pressed coconut oil
- 1 tbsp. swerve
- 1 tbsp. vanilla extract
- ½ tsp sea salt
- 3 tbsp. organic unsweetened cocoa powder

Nutritional Values

- ✓ Calories: 76 kcal
- ✓ Fat: 8g (90%)
- ✓ Carbohydrates: 2.45g (5%)
- ✓ Protein: 1g (5%)
- ✓ Dietary Fiber : 1g
- ✓ Cholesterol: 73mg

How to Make the Dessert

- ➢ Combine the ingredients in a bowl
- ➢ Mix until smooth
- ➢ Drop by tablespoon onto a parchment paper
- ➢ Refrigerate until candies solidify.
- ➢ Store in a covered container in the fridge.

Mint Fudge

Easy to prepare and a healthy dessert choice.

Portion

This recipe serves 4 persons.

Total Time

20 minutes

Ingredients

- 2 tbsp. vanilla extract
- 1 tsp peppermint extract
- 1½ cup pumpkin seeds
- ½ cup dried parsley flakes
- 1 cup cold pressed coconut oil
- ¼ tbsp. sea salt
- ½ cup of swerve

Nutritional Values

- ✓ Calories: 119kcal
- ✓ Fat: 9g (66.9%)
- ✓ Carbohydrates: 9.5g (19.8%)
- ✓ Protein: 4g (13.2%)
- ✓ Dietary Fiber : 3.5g
- ✓ Cholesterol: mg

How to Make the Dessert
- ➢ Melt coconut oil in saucepan.

➢ Add all ingredients into blender, follow by the warm coconut oil and blend until smooth.
➢ Pour into a baking pan.
➢ Freeze it for 4 hours.
➢ Retrieve and cut into pieces.
➢ Store in refrigerator to prevent softening.

Keto Avocado Pudding

Avocado Pudding delightful taste with healthy fats.

Portion

This recipe serves 4 persons.

Total Time

20 minutes

Ingredients

- 2 avocados
- 1 tbsp. fresh lime juice
- 400ml organic coconut milk
- 2 tsp organic vanilla extract
- 80 drops stevia
- 1 tbsp. Cacao Nibs

Nutritional Values

- ✓ Calories: 292kcal
- ✓ Fat: 28.8g (91%)
- ✓ Carbohydrates: 3.8g (6%)
- ✓ Protein: 2.7g (3%)
- ✓ Dietary Fiber : 0g
- ✓ Cholesterol: 0mg

How to Make the Dessert

- ➢ Peeled, pitted and slice the avocado into pieces
- ➢ Add the ingredients into a blender
- ➢ Blend until smooth. Sprinkle cacao nibs on top.
- ➢ Serve it.

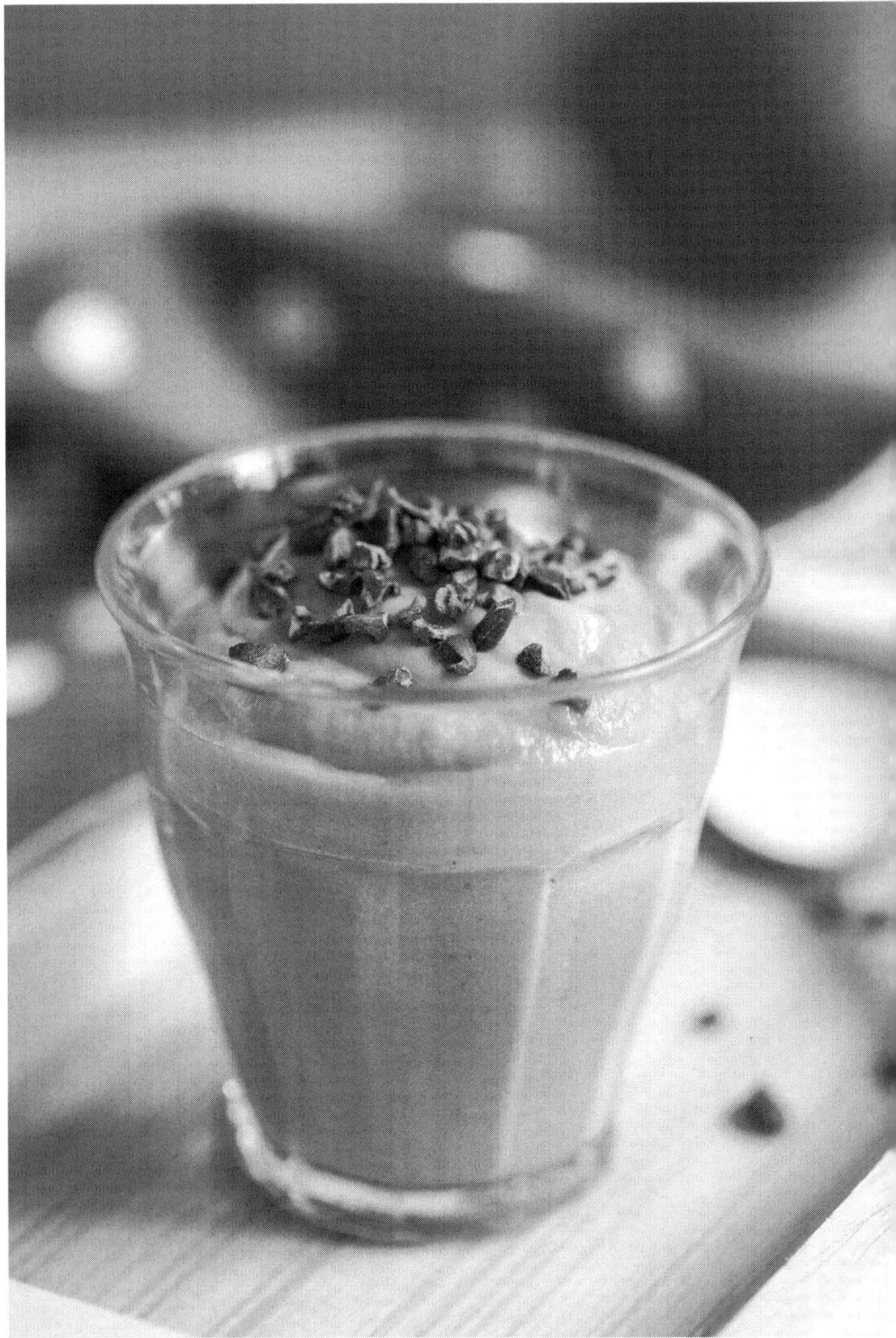

Coconut Pudding

Coconut pudding, your source of healthy saturated fatty acids.

Portion

This recipe serves 2 persons.

Total Time

30 minutes

Ingredients

- 1½ coconut milk
- 1 tbsp. beef gelatin
- 3 egg yolks
- ½ tsp vanilla extract
- 6 tbsp. stevia

Nutritional Values

- ✓ Calories: 291kcal
- ✓ Fat: 8.8g (27%)
- ✓ Carbohydrates: 45g (63%)
- ✓ Protein: 7.6g (10%)
- ✓ Dietary Fiber : 1.8g
- ✓ Cholesterol: 15mg

How to Make the Dessert

- ➢ Mix the gelatin and 1 tbsp. coconut milk in a small bowl. Set aside.
- ➢ Heat the saucepan and add the remaining coconut milk and stevia.

- ➤ Stir for 3 -5 minutes.
- ➤ Pour the hot coconut milk over the egg yolks and whisk it continuously.
- ➤ Transfer the hot mixture back into a pot and cook for 3 – 4 minutes until thicken.
- ➤ Pour the small bowl of gelatin into the pot and stir well.
- ➤ Pour the mixture evenly into 2 ramekins.
- ➤ Refrigerate it for 3 hours to set it
- ➤ Serve it.

Ginger Spice Cookies

It's cookies time!

Portion

This recipe serves 2 persons.

Total Time

25 minutes

Ingredients

- 1 egg
- 3 tbsp. fresh grated ginger
- 2 tbsp cinnamon powder
- 4 tbsp of stevia
- pinch sea salt
- 2 tbsp. chia seeds
- 2 cups almond nuts
- ¼ tsp nutmeg

Nutritional Values

- ✓ Calories: 95kcal
- ✓ Fat: 8g (85%)
- ✓ Carbohydrates: 2g (5%)
- ✓ Protein: 1g (9%)
- ✓ Dietary Fiber : 1g
- ✓ Cholesterol: 0mg

How to Make the Dessert
- ➢ Preheat oven to 350F

- ➢ Blend almond nuts with chia seeds
- ➢ Mix all the ingredient in large bowl
- ➢ Use a tablespoon to create bite size cookies
- ➢ Roll and flatten it with hands
- ➢ Place the cookies on a baking tray lined with parchment paper
- ➢ Bake at 350F for 15 minutes until golden
- ➢ Serve it.

Cardamon Shortbread Cookies

Delectable cookies with tangerine zest!

Portion

This recipe serves 4 persons.

Total Time

30 minutes

Ingredients

- 2 oz 85% or greater cacao dark chocolate
- 2 cups almond flour
- 6 tbsp. butter
- ¼ tsp ground cardamom
- ¼ tsp clementine zest
- ½ cup swerve

Nutritional Values

- ✓ Calories: 124kcal
- ✓ Fat: 11g (86%)
- ✓ Carbohydrates: 2g (1%)
- ✓ Protein: 4g (13%)
- ✓ Dietary Fiber : 2g
- ✓ Cholesterol: 0mg

How to Make the Dessert

- ➢ Mix the cardamom, zest. melted butter, almond flour and swerve in a bowl until evenly mix.
- ➢ Form into a ball and refrigerate it for 10 minutes.

- ➢ Press between 2 sheets of parchment paper
- ➢ Slice into 16 rectangles.
- ➢ Preheat oven at 350F
- ➢ Bake for 15 minutes in the oven until golden brown.
- ➢ Cool and cut along the line.
- ➢ Melt chocolate into a bowl with microwave for 1 minute, or at 30 seconds interval until the chocolate melt.
- ➢ Dip the shortbread cookies into the melted chocolate
- ➢ Place it on a parchment paper to cool
- ➢ Sprinkle clementine zest before the chocolate harden.
- ➢ Server it.

CONCLUSION

There you have everything you need to know to start the ketogenic diet and start losing weight today. I hope this book inspires you to take control of your health and get on the path to a healthy and better living while at the same time losing weight.

The most important thing you can do now is to stay positive and not give up. All weight loss plans have their ups and downs, and there will be weeks when you will lose more weight than others. Nevertheless, if you stick with the diet and stay on track you are going to lose weight and achieve your ultimate weight loss goal.

I know how hard the struggle can be and I definitely understand there are times when you would like nothing more than to just give up. Regardless, you must ignore the negative feelings and focus on the benefits; press on. I lost the weight I wanted and I am happier and much healthier than I have ever been. Stick with the diet and stay strong and you will be happier and healthier, too.

You deserve to be happy and healthy. With the right tools, you can be both. Follow this advice and make this year a new beginning and a start of the happiest and healthiest time of your life.

Good luck!

NOTES

How does the brain use food as energy? -
http://www.brainfacts.org/about-neuroscience/ask-an-expert/articles/2012/how-does-the-brain-use-food-as-energy/

Each Organ has a Unique Metabolic Profile -
https://www.ncbi.nlm.nih.gov/books/NBK22436/

The Fat-Fueled Brain: Unnatural or Advantageous? -
https://blogs.scientificamerican.com/mind-guest-blog/the-fat-fueled-brain-unnatural-or-advantageous/

Ketogenic Ratio, Calories and Fluids: Do They Matter? -
https://www.ncbi.nlm.nih.gov/pmc/articles/PMC2656445/

Ketogenic Diet for Obesity: Friend or Foe? -
https://www.ncbi.nlm.nih.gov/pmc/articles/PMC3945587/

Long Term Long-term effects of a ketogenic diet in obese patients -
https://www.ncbi.nlm.nih.gov/pmc/articles/PMC2716748/

Mechanism of Ketogenic Diet Action
https://www.ncbi.nlm.nih.gov/books/NBK98219/

Metabolic Effects of the Very-Low-Carbohydrate Diets: Misunderstood "Villains" of Human Metabolism –
https://www.ncbi.nlm.nih.gov/pmc/articles/PMC2129159/

RECIPES INDEX

T

Z

Y

ABOUT THE AUTHOR

Roy Nolan is an avid chef, self-taught nutritionist and wellness enthusiast. His strong passion for healthy living, dieting, nutrition and weight loss leads to his successful transformation. He is an entrepreneur, a fitness buff and a part-time author.

Since childhood, Roy, a young growing boy has a huge appetite, especially during his teenage years. His weight begun to balloon quickly and by the age of 18, he was already 120kg.

Roy hates looking at himself in the mirror. He decided to put an end to it and love himself. Like everyone, he looked for an easy way out and tried almost every type of diet pills to be skinny again. But none of it worked and worst some of the pills induced terrible side effects.

Eventually, Roy realized that this is a vicious cycle and is not a long-term solution. Roy started to learn about the potential benefits of diets such as Paleo, Atkins & Ketogenic and decided that Ketogenic diet could be the answer to his problem.

Today, his successful transformation was made possible with years of research (since 2006) and applying the right actions.

Roy decided to compile and share his knowledge of different diets in some of the books he has written.

In his spare time, Roy likes to hit the gym and participate in runs.

Did you like this book?

If you would like to read more great books like this one, why not subscribe to our website and receive <u>LIFETIME Updates</u> on all our latest promotions, upcoming books and new book releases, and free books or gifts that we occasionally pamper our loyal members.

https://goo.gl/fDhJLm

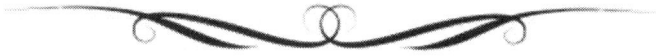

Check out Roy's other proud works below if you didn't get a chance or follow Roy at
https://goo.gl/hU7QZD

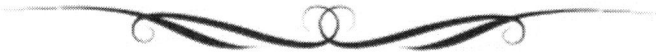

Thanks for reading! Please add a short review on Amazon and let me know what your thoughts! - Roy

PAVO PRESS

We would like to thank you again for reading this book. Lots of effort, planning and time were committed to ensure that you are receiving the best possible information with as much value as possible. We hope you have unlocked the values from this book.

If you've feel that you have benefited and find that this book is helpful, we would like to ask for a small favor.

Please kindly leave a positive review on Amazon or your favorite social media.

Your review is appreciated and will go a long way to motivate us in producing more quality books for your reading pleasure and needs.

- END -

Made in the USA
Lexington, KY
06 July 2018